Contemporary Diagnosis and Management of The Hypertensive Patient®

Matthew R. Weir, MD
Professor and Director
Division of Nephrology
University of Maryland School of Medicine, Baltimore

Domenic A. Sica, MD
Professor, Department of Internal Medicine and Pharmacology
Chairman, Section of Clinical Pharmacology and Hypertension,
Division of Nephrology,
Virginia Commonwealth University, Richmond

First Edition

Published by Handbooks in Health Care Co.,
Newtown, Pennsylvania, USA

This book has been prepared and is presented as a service to the medical community. The information provided reflects the knowledge, experience, and personal opinions of Matthew R. Weir, MD, Professor and Director, Division of Nephrology, University of Maryland School of Medicine, Baltimore, and Domenic A. Sica, MD, Professor, Department of Internal Medicine and Pharmacology, and Chairman, Section of Clinical Pharmacology and Hypertension, Division of Nephrology, Virginia Commonwealth University, Richmond.

This book is not intended to replace or to be used as a substitute for the complete prescribing information prepared by each manufacturer for each drug. Because of possible variations in drug indications, in dosage information, in newly described toxicities, in drug/drug interactions, and in other items of importance, reference to such complete prescribing information is definitely recommended before any of the drugs discussed are used or prescribed.

International Standard Book Number: 978-1-931981-81-1

Library of Congress Catalog Card Number: 2008920459

Table of Contents

Foreword

Contemporary Diagnosis and Management of the Hypertensive Patient® by Drs. Matthew R. Weir and Domenic A. Sica is a valuable addition to the sources of information about hypertension, the most common reason that Americans see a clinician. It has 16 brief chapters, eight written by each co-author. Each chapter represents the author's personal opinion on issues facing the practicing clinician, who is likely to have to manage dozens of hypertensive patients each month.

The handbook covers a range of practice-based topics, including how to set goals for treatment, an update on the latest clinical trials, treatment options for special populations, and timely management issues, such as for patients with sleep apnea and for the hypertensive athlete. There are comprehensive chapters on the major drug classes used to treat hypertension, on combination therapy, and on the use of nonsteroidal anti-inflammatory agents.

While this book is targeted to the primary care clinician, some of the chapters go into considerable depth, making it valuable to the specialist as well. It is full of practice "pearls," experienced-based tips on how to manage problems confronting the hypertensive patient, and it has the instructive approach of first asking and then answering Frequently Asked Questions (FAQs).

The suggested readings at the end of each chapter give the reader the basis for the opinion of the author who has posed and answered the questions, in case the reader disagrees with the author, something that is inevitable in medicine. Although there are now numerous internet sources of information, this book easily fits into a laboratory coat pocket and can provide useful advice as fast as it takes to search on-line.

Henry Black, MD
Clinical Professor of Internal Medicine,
Director of Hypertension Research,
New York University School of Medicine,
NYU Center for the Prevention
of Cardiovascular Disease,
New York, NY

Chapter 1

How to Set Blood-Pressure Goals

Blood pressure increases as we age. However, it does so at a variable rate. It is likely that the increasing slope of blood pressure over time is associated with the increased risk of vascular disease. Regardless of age, there is a continuous relationship between blood pressure and cardiovascular events. As a result, it is important to identify patients who are at risk for an earlier and steeper blood-pressure slope so that appropriate management strategies can be implemented. It is likely that genetic factors control the blood-pressure slope, which may be related to subtle changes in sodium and water handling by the kidneys and/or changes in hormonal factors that regulate blood pressure. Consequently, setting individual blood-pressure goals is an important issue.

Many committees that establish hypertension treatment guidelines are moving away from threshold treatment recommendations and more toward global cardiovascular risk assessment with individualized choices for blood-pressure goals. This approach is based on epidemiologic observations indicating that earlier management and lower blood-pressure goals often provide more opportunity for cardiovascular risk reduction. Older guidelines suggested that treatment be delayed until certain blood-pressure thresholds are reached. Unfortunately, this traditional approach often delays therapeutic intervention, so many patients require later-stage treatment that often requires the use of multiple drugs.

Frequently Asked Questions

1. Aside from traditional Framingham Heart Study (FHS) risk factors, what are the newer ways of assessing cardiovascular risk?

It is important to realize that classic risk factors should always be considered as part of a cardiovascular risk evaluation: male gender, age >50 years, hypertension, diabetes, high cholesterol, cigarette smoking, sedentary lifestyle, obesity. However, it is also critically important to obtain a detailed family history from the patient. This is often overlooked and is one of the most powerful tools for assessing timing and risk for cardiovascular events. In addition to these understandings, more sensitive screening for the presence or absence of diabetes is essential. Type 2 diabetes often requires many years to clinically manifest. Patients typically progress from impaired fasting glucose (IFG) to impaired glucose tolerance (IGT) to clinical diabetes. Earlier identification of glycemic abnormalities may assist in the quicker recognition of a patient at increased risk of cardiovascular events, and appropriate implementation of lower blood-pressure goals, preferably <130/80 mm Hg. In large part, this blood-pressure recommendation is based on the results of the Hypertension Optimal Treatment (HOT) study. The primary focus of the HOT study was reducing diastolic blood pressure to levels <80 mm Hg. Although only about 8% of nearly 20,000 participants in this study were diabetic, it was evident that those diabetics who achieved a diastolic blood-pressure goal <80 mm Hg were least likely to experience cardiovascular events. The secondary evaluation of systolic blood pressure from the HOT study also indicated that a blood-pressure goal <130 mm Hg was optimal in diabetics. Although the guidelines committees recommend a blood-pressure goal <130/80 mm Hg, even lower goals in some diabetics could potentially be advantageous. Currently, there are studies under way to evaluate the potential benefit of achieving a systolic blood pressure <120 mm Hg in diabetics.

Another important means of assessing cardiovascular risk is to establish a patient's estimated glomerular filtration rate (eGFR) and screen quantitatively for protein in the urine. It is evident from epidemiologic studies that patients with equation-based eGFR <60 mL/min/1.73 m^2 are at increased risk for cardiovascular events. Likewise, there is a continuous relationship between the amount of albumin or protein in the urine and risk for cardiovascular events. As such, blood-pressure guidelines committees have listed an eGFR <60 mL/min/1.73 m^2 and microalbuminuria at 30 mg albumin/g/creatinine as coronary artery disease (CAD) equivalents and a recommended blood-pressure treatment goal of <130/80 mm Hg.

Using established FHS risk factors, a detailed family history, and objective screening for abnormalities of glycemic control (ie, fasting plasma glucose [FPG], 2-hour postprandial glucose, hemoglobin A_{1c} [HbA_{1c}] and equation-based GFR assessment or spot quantitation of a urine albumin-to-creatinine ratio can assist in evaluating CAD risk and provide a more objective means for setting appropriate blood-pressure goals.

2. How do you set blood-pressure goals for older patients? Should this be different compared with younger patients?

The age of the patient should play a role in the decision-making process to set blood-pressure treatment goals. Younger patients have intact baroreceptor reflexes and are thus more likely to tolerate lower blood-pressure goals. But older patients may have greater susceptibility to orthostatic changes in blood pressure with treatment. For patients >55 years, systolic blood pressure is the major therapeutic target because it correlates more accurately with CAD risk than does diastolic blood pressure. Systolic blood pressure is usually more difficult to treat. Some of the difficulty in treating elevated levels of systolic blood pressure is related to the impaired vasorelaxation response of vessels that are thickened and calcified and have lost much of their elasticity and normal endothelial responses. Despite this, systolic blood pressure in older patients can be controlled with the careful use of drugs that work well with one another.

In younger patients, diastolic blood pressure is the principal target. The diastolic blood pressure often responds more easily to conventional treatment in younger patients than in older patients with isolated systolic hypertension. It is important to note that there are no data to suggest that a patient's age should influence the setting of blood-pressure goals. The data from the treatment trials of isolated systolic hypertension in older patients indicate that, to prevent cardiovascular events, an intermediate systolic blood-pressure goal <160 mm Hg is appropriate, with a long-term goal of approximately 140 mm Hg. Moreover, the Hypertension in the Very Elderly Trial (HYVET) which assessed the effect of a diuretic (sustained-release indapamide 2.5 mg) and an angiotensin-converting enzyme (ACE) inhibitor (perindopril [Aceon®] 2 or 4 mg) vs placebo in elderly individuals (ie, >80 years) with systolic predominant hypertension, found that a target blood pressure of <150/80 mm Hg could be reached (starting blood pressure 173/90/8 mm Hg with a mean blood-pressure reduction of 15/6.1 mm Hg), with a 30% reduction in rate of fatal and nonfatal stroke, and a 64% reduction in the rate of heart failure.

3. *Is there a J-shape curve for lowering blood pressure?*

In older patients, there is a concern that, as one sets lower systolic blood-pressure treatment goals, the associated reduction in diastolic blood pressure could increase the risk for cardiovascular events. This is important because it raises the issue that there may be a J-shape curve in setting lower systolic blood-pressure goals in older patients. Unfortunately, clinical trial data are not clear about whether a J-shape curve actually exists. Often, it is difficult to accurately measure diastolic blood pressure in people who have a high systolic blood pressure. In addition, the diastolic blood pressure often drops to a much smaller degree than the systolic blood pressure during treatment. There are also few patients in clinical trials who reach a diastolic blood pressure <60 mm Hg.

4. Are patients with faster heart rates more susceptible to the effects of lower diastolic blood pressure?

The majority of coronary artery perfusions occurs during diastole, thus patients with faster heart rates could be more susceptible to ischemia, particularly if they have a lower diastolic blood pressure. More studies need to carefully evaluate this concern, particularly in older patients with faster heart rates and low diastolic blood pressure.

5. Are other demographic factors important as you set blood-pressure goals?

There is no available information to suggest that gender, ethnicity, or body mass index (BMI) should alter decisions when setting a patient's blood-pressure goals. Rather than considering demographic factors, the clinician should focus on the estimation of cardiovascular risk with the FHS score and on the objective measures of glycemic control and kidney function.

6. Is home blood-pressure monitoring of use in the treatment of hypertension ?

Conventional office blood-pressure measurement yields higher blood-pressure values than home-based readings, particularly for systolic blood pressure. The level of home blood pressure suggested to best correspond to a normal clinic blood pressure of 140/90 mm Hg is about 135/85 mm Hg. Home blood-pressure monitoring provides a large number of readings, and, thus, in a given patient, adds to the precision of blood-pressure determination over time.

Home blood-pressure monitoring is useful for the long-term follow-up of patients with white-coat hypertension and the evaluation of treatment efficacy in patients with sustained hypertension. Technical, economic, and behavioral barriers have until now impeded the widespread use of home monitoring in clinical practice. The number of clinic visits may be reduced with home blood-pressure monitoring, making it a potentially cost-effective means for the management of hypertensive patients. Studies have shown that adjustment of antihypertensive therapy based on home blood pressure instead of office blood pressure leads to less intensive drug therapy. Although home blood-pressure monitoring still requires further validation, it is increasingly viewed as an important component of the treatment plan for the patient with hypertension.

Suggested Readings

Beckett NS, Peters R, Fletcher AE, et al, and the HYVET Study Group: Treatment of hypertension in patients 80 years of age or older. *N Engl J Med* 2008;358:1887-1898.

Chobanian AV, Bakris GL, Black HR, et al: The Seventh Report of the Joint National Committee on Prevention, Detection, Evaluation, and Treatment of High Blood Pressure: the JNC 7 report. *JAMA* 2003;289:2560-2572; erratum *JAMA* 2003;290:197.

Giles TD, Berk BC, Black HR, et al: Expanding the definition and classification of hypertension. *J Clin Hypertens (Greenwich)* 2005;7:505-512.

Greenlund KJ, Croft JB, Mensah GA: Prevalence of heart disease and stroke risk factors in persons with prehypertension in the United States, 1999-2000. *Arch Intern Med* 2004;164:2113-2118.

Hansson L, Zanchetti A, Carruthers SG, et al: Effects of intensive blood-pressure lowering and low-dose aspirin in patients with hypertension: principal results of the Hypertension Optimal Treatment (HOT) randomised trial. HOT Study Group. *Lancet* 1998;351: 1755-1762.

Kshirsagar AV, Carpenter M, Bang H, et al: Blood pressure usually considered normal is associated with an elevated risk of cardiovascular disease. *Am J Med* 2006;119:133-141.

Lewington S, Clarke R, Qizilbash N, et al: Age-specific relevance of usual blood pressure to vascular mortality: a meta-analysis of individual data for one million adults in 61 prospective studies. *Lancet* 2002;360:1903-1913; erratum *Lancet* 2003;361:1060.

Mancia G, De Backer G, Dominiczak A, et al: 2007 Guidelines for the Management of Arterial Hypertension: The Task Force for the Management of Arterial Hypertension of the European Society of Hypertension (ESH) and of the European Society of Cardiology (ESC). *J Hypertens* 2007;25:1105-1187; erratum *J Hypertens* 2007;25:1105-1187.

Pickering TG, Miller NH, Ogedegbe G, et al: Call to action on use and reimbursement for home blood pressure monitoring: executive summary: a joint scientific statement from the American Heart Association, American Society Of Hypertension, and Preventive Cardiovascular Nurses Association. *Hypertension* 2008;52:1-9.

Rosamond W, Flegal K, Friday G, et al: Heart disease and stroke statistics—2007 update: a report from the American Heart Association Statistics Committee and Stroke Statistics Subcommittee. *Circulation* 2007;115:e69-e171; erratum *Circulation* 2007;115:e172.

Sarnak MJ, Levey AS, Schoolwerth AC, et al: Kidney disease as a risk factor for development of cardiovascular disease: a statement from the American Heart Association Councils on Kidney in Cardiovascular Disease, High Blood Pressure Research, Clinical Cardiology, and Epidemiology and Prevention. *Hypertension* 2003;42:1050-1065.

Vasan RS, Larson MG, Leip EP, et al: Impact of high-normal blood pressure on the risk of cardiovascular disease. *N Engl J Med* 2001; 345:1291-1297.

Weycker D, Nichols GA, O'Keeffe-Rosetti M, et al: Risk-factor clustering and cardiovascular disease risk in hypertensive patients. *Am J Hypertens* 2007;20:599-607.

Chapter **2**

Recent Clinical Trials in Hypertension—Lessons Learned

A number of important clinical trials in hypertension have been completed and published in the past 5 to 7 years. These trials have improved our understanding of hypertension in terms of optimal blood-pressure goals and treatment measures, cardiovascular and renal disease end points, and surrogate measures of benefit, ie, preventing new-onset diabetes, reducing the likelihood of congestive heart failure (CHF), regressing left-ventricular hypertrophy (LVH), and albuminuria. These clinical trials demonstrate that the prompt control of blood pressure, the lowering of blood pressure, and modifying the activity of the renin-angiotensin-aldosterone system (RAAS) provides incremental opportunities to prevent cardiovascular events and renal disease progression. However, many important questions remain to be answered.

The Heart Outcomes Protection Evaluation (HOPE) study examined the 4- to 5-year outcomes of >9,000 66-year-old patients with known cardiovascular disease (CVD) risk factors or with evident CVD. These patients were randomized to receive either the angiotensin-converting enzyme (ACE) inhibitor ramipril (Altace®) (10 mg) or placebo in addition to their existing medical regimen. The primary outcome of the HOPE study was a composite of myocardial infarction (MI), stroke, or death from any cardiovascular cause. The majority of patients in the trial were on antihypertensive medications, which primarily included calcium-channel blockers (CCBs) and β-blockers before randomization. At the time of randomization, mean blood pressure was 139/79 mm Hg, which indicates that these patients had blood-pressure levels that would be appropriate according to current guidelines. Patients receiving additional ACE inhibitor therapy experienced a 3 to 10 mm Hg further reduction in systolic blood pressure during follow-up, depending upon whether casual blood-pressure readings were used, or a subset of patients who had 24-hour ambulatory blood-pressure monitoring. Patients in the ACE inhibitor arm of the trial experienced a 22% reduction in cardiovascular end points, which was in part due to the lower blood pressure achieved, but perhaps also due to the incremental benefit of RAAS inhibition. In addition, these patients experienced less progression of albuminuria, less new-onset diabetes, and less new presentation of congestive heart failure (CHF).

In the Antihypertensive and Lipid-Lowering Treatment to Prevent Heart Attack Trial (ALLHAT), >33,000 patients were randomized into a three-arm trial (after the doxazosin [Cardura®] arm was terminated) to evaluate whether monotherapy with either a diuretic, a CCB, or an ACE inhibitor would be more effective in preventing cardiovascular events. The majority of patients entering the trial had a blood pressure of approximately 145/83 mm Hg and were typically on one medication. After removal of that medication, they were randomized to receive amlodipine (Norvasc®), chlorthalidone or lisinopril (Prinivil®, Zestril®). Additional medications could be added to achieve a blood pressure <140/90 mm Hg. The primary outcome over the 5 years of the trial was fatal or nonfatal MI. The ALLHAT participants were similar demographically to the patients in the HOPE study with regard to age and concurrent diabetes. However, ALLHAT had greater ethnic minority representation. A mean number of two medications were used to control blood pressure in

ALLHAT. Unlike the clinical trial design in the HOPE study, in which the RAAS-blocking regimen had a blood-pressure advantage, ALLHAT's thiazide diuretic and CCB arms had a substantial blood-pressure advantage over the lisinopril regimen. Despite these blood-pressure differences, cumulative event rates for all three therapies were not different for the primary outcome. However, there were fewer strokes in the chlorthalidone-treated patients and less heart failure in the chlorthalidone- and ACE inhibitor-based regimens. New-onset diabetes was less common in the ACE inhibitor arm of ALLHAT, compared with the thiazide diuretic and CCB arms.

In the Valsartan Antihypertensive Longitudinal Use Evaluation (VALUE) study, >15,000 patients were randomized to receive either an angiotensin-receptor blocker (ARB)-based regimen (valsartan [Diovan®]) compared with a CCB-based regimen (amlodipine) to lower blood pressure over the course of 5 years. All patients could receive additional medications to lower blood pressure to <140/90 mm Hg, if the primary therapies did not achieve blood-pressure control. The additional medications were primarily thiazide diuretics or β-blockers. In the VALUE study, the participants had a mean age of 67 years and approximately one third had prestudy evidence of diabetes. During follow-up, the amlodipine regimen had an early 2 to 4 mm Hg blood-pressure advantage over the valsartan regimen. Despite this blood-pressure difference, there was no difference in the primary composite cardiac end point. Perhaps the most important observation in the VALUE study was that early control of blood pressure with a CCB-based regimen provided an important opportunity to reduce the risk of cardiovascular events in the first 6 months of the study. Fewer patients in the ARB arm developed heart failure or new-onset diabetes compared with the CCB arm.

The Losartan Intervention for End Point Reduction in Hypertension (LIFE) study evaluated the effects of either an ARB-based regimen (losartan [Cozaar®]) or β-blocker-based regimen (atenolol [Tenormin®]) on cardiovascular outcomes in >9,000 people with hypertension and LVH. Per protocol, thiazide diuretics could be added along with other medications to facilitate the achievement of a blood-pressure level <140/90 mm Hg. The primary end point of this study was cardiovascular morbidity and mortality. During follow-up, despite nearly identical reductions in blood pressure in the two arms, there was a 13% reduction in the risk of primary composite cardiac end point in the ARB regimen compared with the β-blocker regimen. The majority of the cardiovascular risk reduction was related to a 25% reduction in stroke in the ARB arm. There was also a more effective regression of LVH in the ARB arm as well as less new-onset diabetes compared with the β-blocker arm. Of additional interest, in this study was a secondary analysis showing that not only was baseline albuminuria predictive of cardiovascular events, but so was time-varying albuminuria during follow-up. There were no absolute differences in the incidence of MI between the two groups, indicating that both therapeutic strategies were similarly effective as part of an effective blood-pressure-lowering regimen.

The Anglo-Scandinavian Cardiac Outcome Trial (ASCOT) randomized >19,000 people to receive two different blood-pressure-lowering regimens that incorporated either a β-blocker and a thiazide diuretic, or a CCB and an ACE inhibitor for 5 years. The primary end point of the trial was nonfatal MI and fatal coronary disease. Although there was no difference in the primary outcome between the two groups, this trial was terminated early because of the significant overall cardiovascular benefits in the CCB/ACE inhibitor arm (amlodipine [Norvasc®]/perindopril [Aceon®]) compared with the β-blocker/thiazide diuretic (atenolol/bendroflumethiazide) arm. The CCB/ACE inhibitor regimen also had a blood-pressure-lowering advantage of almost 3 mm Hg for the first two years of the study. However, this advantage narrowed during the 5 years of follow-up. Overall, there was a 25% reduction in cardiovascular mortality and a 30% reduction in the incidence of new-onset diabetes in the CCB/ACE inhibitor arm. A subset of ASCOT patients also participated in a study to evaluate the measurement of central aortic pressures as a predictor of cardiovascular outcome. In this substudy, a robust reduction in central aortic pressures associated with the CCB/ACE inhibitor regimen were predictive of an improved cardiovascular outcome despite the fact that cuff blood-pressure differences between the two groups were not present.

Frequently Asked Questions

1. In these large clinical trials, how many antihypertensive medications were required for patients to achieve an appropriate blood-pressure goal?

In general, the participants in these studies were in their late 50s or 60s and often had substantial medical comorbidities, ie, diabetes, dyslipidemia, a prior history of CVD. Typically, the participants took between two and four drugs to lower blood pressure. In addition, these patients often required multiple other medications. These large clinical trials indicated that, if patients could remain compliant with the blood-pressure-lowering regimens, blood-pressure levels would improve for most of them with a significant attenuation of cardiovascular event rates.

2. What were the best antihypertensive medications to lower blood pressure in these studies?

Every patient is different. It is apparent from these studies that, given the age, weight, and overall health of the patients studied, the use of thiazide diuretics or CCBs provided important early opportunities to control blood pressure. However, equally as important were the advantages of RAAS blockade to help facilitate blood-pressure reduction in concert with these drugs. Because the majority of patients required two or more medications, it is not surprising that patients who received either a thiazide diuretic or a CCB in conjunction with a RAAS blocker not only achieved better blood-pressure reduction but also experienced fewer cardiovascular events and less progression of surrogate measures of outcome. Ultimately, the choice of drugs to lower blood pressure needs to be individualized for each patient based on efficacy and tolerability.

3. Should everyone who requires antihypertensive medication be prescribed a drug that modifies RAAS activity?

The results obtained from these large trials indicate that patients with risk factors for or with evident CVD or renal disease can achieve important benefits from using drugs that block the RAAS as part of an effective blood-pressure-lowering regimen. However, not every patient can tolerate these drugs. Moreover, RAAS inhibitors should be used cautiously in females of childbearing age because they are contraindicated in the second and third trimesters of pregnancy. These drugs also have important opportunities for both renal and cardiovascular protection; however, they are not a substitute for achieving appropriate blood-pressure goals.

4. Are ARBs and ACE inhibitors of similar capability in providing cardiovascular protection?

It is apparent from the results of these large trials that both lower blood pressure and blocking the RAAS provide important opportunities for reducing the risk of cardiovascular events. However, one must also respect the fact that these drugs do have somewhat different mechanisms of action, which could in the long term prove to be either beneficial (or detrimental) with regard to cardiovascular events. In one large noninferiority trial of 15,000 post-MI patients, the ACE inhibitor captopril (Capoten®) was compared with the ARB valsartan (Diovan®). Both regimens were similarly successful in reducing the incidence of cardiovascular events. This trial illustrates the cardioprotective similarity between these drug classes.

5. Are ARBs more effective than ACE inhibitors in reducing the incidence of stroke?

This is an important question because available clinical trial evidence does support the conclusion that ARBs provide an important opportunity to reduce stroke as part of an effective blood-pressure-lowering regimen. The results of clinical trials with ACE inhibitors are not as conclusive, but this does not mean that ACE inhibitors are not effective. It just means that they have not been adequately tested (perhaps in the right doses) to answer this question. Given that ARBs do possess the advantage of reducing the potential of suffering a stroke, they may be the preferred therapy to prevent recurrent stroke compared with an ACE inhibitor.

6. Does preventing new-onset diabetes with drugs that block the RAAS prevent cardiovascular death?

No trials discussed in this handbook provide evidence that preventing new-onset diabetes is associated with a reduction of cardiovascular end points. The potential benefit of preventing new-onset diabetes in limiting the subsequent risk for cardiovascular events is theoretical. However, epidemiologic evidence indicates that diabetes is associated with an increased risk for cardiovascular events. Perhaps this may prove to be an important intermediate measure of benefit. The clinical trial evidence indicating that RAAS blockers can prevent new-onset diabetes in hypertensive patients on medication is quite consistent regardless of concomitant therapies and is the case in about 25% of the patients studied.

Suggested Readings

ALLHAT Officers and Coordinators for the ALLHAT Collaborative Research Group. The Antihypertensive and Lipid-Lowering Treatment to Prevent Heart Attack Trial: Major outcomes in high-risk hypertensive patients randomized to angiotensin-converting enzyme inhibitor or calcium channel blocker vs diuretic: The Antihypertensive and Lipid-Lowering Treatment to Prevent Heart Attack Trial (ALLHAT). *JAMA* 2002;288:2981-2997.

Andraws R, Brown DL: Effect of inhibition of the renin-angiotensin system on development of type 2 diabetes mellitus (meta-analysis of randomized trials). *Am J Cardiol* 2007;99:1006-1012.

Bangalore S, Parkar S. Grossman E, et al: A meta-analysis of 94,492 patients with hypertension treated with beta blockers to determine the risk of new-onset diabetes mellitus. *Am J Cardiol* 2007; 100:1254-1262.

Dahlof B, Devereux RB, Kjeldsen SE, et al, and the LIFE Study Group: Cardiovascular morbidity and mortality in the Losartan Intervention For Endpoint reduction in hypertension study (LIFE): a randomised trial against atenolol. *Lancet* 2002;359:995-1003.

Julius S, Kjeldsen SE, Weber M, et al: Outcomes in hypertensive patients at high cardiovascular risk treated with regimens based on valsartan or amiodipine; the VALUE randomised trial. *Lancet* 2004; 363;2022-2031.

McMurray J, Solomon S, Pieper K, et al: The effect of valsartan, captopril, or both on atherosclerotic events after acute myocardial infarction: an analysis of the Valsartan in Acute Myocardial Infarction Trial (VALIANT). *J Am Coll Cardiol* 2006;47:726-733.

Sever PS, Dahlof B, Poulter NR, et al: Rationale, design, methods and baseline demography of participants of the Anglo-Scandinavian Cardiac Outcomes Trial. ASCOT investigators. *J Hypertens* 2001;19: 1139-1147.

Verma S, Mamdani MM, Al-Omran M, et al: Angiotensin receptor blockers vs. angiotensin converting enzyme inhibitors and acute coronary syndrome outcomes in elderly patients; a population-based cohort study (UMPIRE study results). *JASH* 2007;1:286-294.

Weir MR: Providing end-organ protection with renin-angiotensin system inhibition: the evidence so far. *J Clin Hypertens (Greenwich)* 2006;8:99-105.

Yusuf S, Sleight P, Pogue J, et al: Effects of an angiotensin-converting-enzyme inhibitor, ramipril, on cardiovascular events in high-risk patients. The Heart Outcomes Prevention Evaluation Study Investigators. *N Engl J Med* 2000;342:145-153.

Chapter 3

Sleep Apnea and Hypertension

Significant research has focused on the link between sleep apnea and hypertension, and the evidence suggesting an association between these two conditions is persuasive. Sleep apnea is common, easily diagnosed, and very treatable. Sleep apnea syndromes consist of two related disorders, obstructive sleep apnea (OSA), which is more common, and central sleep apnea (CSA). The estimated prevalence of OSA is 2% in women and 4% in the adult male population. It has a greater prevalence in young blacks (<25 years) than in whites, and is also more prevalent in the aged. More than 50% of individuals with OSA are found to have hypertension based on office blood-pressure readings. This number would be considerably higher if ambulatory blood-pressure monitoring were to be used to determine blood-pressure load.

Obesity is so widespread in OSA that the index of suspicion for this disease should be high in any hypertensive patient with a body mass index (BMI) >27 kg/m^2. In patients with higher BMIs, OSA occurs because of anatomic changes favoring repetitive episodes of upper airway occlusion during inspiration. In this regard, sleep onset is followed by a reduction in neural drive to the muscles responsible for maintaining patency of the upper airway, rendering the airway more collapsible.

Any hypertensive patient (with new onset or worsening of existing status of the condition) should be methodically questioned for symptoms of OSA, including snoring, witnessed apnea, irregular breathing during sleep, restless sleeping, chronic morning fatigue, frequent traffic accidents, and declining cognitive function. Often it is the sleep partner who provides the most dependable history, especially on the subject of snoring, because the affected individual often is unaware of the problem. Of note, even habitual snorers without a clinically relevant increase in nocturnal apneas have a higher incidence rate of hypertension. If the diagnosis of OSA is suspected based on clinical grounds and resistant hypertension is present, a formal sleep study may provide added direction to hypertension therapy.

While obesity is known to be an important contributor to OSA, patients with OSA may independently be at risk for further weight gain; conversely, treatment of OSA can reduce body and visceral fat buildup, but somewhat unreliably so. In this regard, patients with newly diagnosed OSA often have a recent history of excessive weight gain in the weeks to months prior to diagnosis. The mechanisms of this weight gain are multifactorial and consist of a more sedentary lifestyle because of daytime somnolence as well as resistance to the appetite suppressant and metabolic effects of leptin. Poorer sleep quality with fragmentation and shorter sleep periods may have a reinforcing role in fatigue and daytime somnolence.

Even modest weight loss (approximately 10 kg) improves sleep apnea, and successful gastric bypass surgery may lead to complete resolution of OSA. Sustained and effective treatment of OSA with continuous positive airway pressure (CPAP) has been reported to lower nighttime and daytime blood pressure in hypertensive patients with OSA and may also improve cardiac ischemia and heart failure symptoms. By reducing apnea/hypopnea frequency and intensity, acute CPAP therapy also minimizes sympathetic nervous system (SNS) activation, which prompts nocturnal blood-pressure surges.

CPAP is usually delivered by a tightly fitted nasal mask. Pressures of 10 to 15 mm Hg are typically required to eradicate snoring, apneas, and hypopneas, as well as episodic desaturation. Compliance (somewhat arbitrarily defined as use for ≥4 hours on ≥5 nights/week) remains the most difficult part of CPAP treatment, with only about 50% to 60% of patients complying with their prescribed CPAP dose. Improvements in the quality of sleep in OSA patients can also occur as a result of a variety of positioning measures during sleep, particularly sleeping on one's side. The role of oral prostheses and surgical approaches needs to be more completely defined. Typically, such devices advance the mandible and thrust the tongue forward, lessening the opportunity for airway closure.

CPAP often fails to completely correct the hypertensive state, so antihypertensive therapy remains necessary. No specific class of antihypertensive drugs has been proven superior for blood-pressure lowering in OSA patients. Medications that cause sedation or increase daytime somnolence should be avoided in the patient with OSA. Such is the case with clonidine (Catapres®), which is a common add-on therapy for the treatment of hypertension in the patient with OSA.

Frequently Asked Questions

1. What are the mechanisms causing hypertension in the patient with OSA?

The association between obesity and hypertension is unequivocal, having been demonstrated in large population studies, and presents as a direct linear relationship between BMI and blood pressure. Because obesity and OSA often coexist, it is likely that OSA plays a meaningful role (as well as the converse for obesity and OSA) in obesity-related hypertension. In addition, daytime blood-pressure values closely correlate with the level of overnight desaturation as well as the number of apnea/hypopnea episodes that occur while the patient is asleep. For example, the odds ratio (OR) is 2.89 for the occurrence of hypertension with a baseline apnea/hypopnea index (AHI) of >15 events/hour. Hypoxemia, hypercarbia, and arousal from sleep repetitively occur with the apnea/hypopnea episodes characteristic of OSA. This sequence of events restricts the natural fall in blood pressure and heart rate when asleep, and based on the frequency/intensity of apnea/hypopnea, episodes will variably affect daytime blood-pressure values in the patient with OSA. The increase in nocturnal blood pressure in patients with OSA can be abrupt and sometimes quite significant.

The mechanism by which OSA causes hypertension is multifactorial, with nocturnal and daytime residual SNS activation being key factors. In addition, sodium retention occurs in obesity (and probably sleep apnea)-induced hypertension in association with activation of the renin-angiotensin-aldosterone system (RAAS) (elevated levels of angiotensin II [Ang II] and plasma aldosterone are often present) and SNS (baroreflex and chemoreflex dysfunction) and through elevated leptin levels. Hyperleptinemia may provide a broader link between OSA and hypertension because leptin may increase adrenergic activity per se, which as previously mentioned is an important determinant of hypertension in OSA.

Increased oxidative stress, endothelial dysfunction, elevated plasma-aldosterone concentrations, and vascular remodeling have also been implicated in obesity and OSA-related hypertension. In obese patients, endothelial dysfunction can reduce vasodilator potential via either enhanced endothelin production or a reduction in nitric oxide (NO) production (NO levels increase with CPAP in patients with OSA).

2. Do ACE inhibitors have a role in the treatment of OSA-related hypertension?

There have been few head-to-head studies that have compared various antihypertensive medication drug classes in the patient with OSA and hypertension. In one of the few comparative therapy studies in patients with hypertension and OSA, the effects of five drug classes (given once daily in the morning) were evaluated through office and ambulatory blood-pressure determinations. The drugs studied were a β-blocker (atenolol [Tenormin®] 50 mg), a calcium-channel blocker (CCB) (amlodipine [Norvasc®] 5 mg), an angiotensin-converting enzyme (ACE) inhibitor (enalapril [Vasotec®] 20 mg), a thiazide diuretic (hydrochlorothiazide [Esidrix®, Microzide®] 25 mg), and an angiotensin-receptor blocker (ARB) (losartan [Cozaar®] 50 mg). Office diastolic blood pressure and mean nighttime ambulatory diastolic and systolic blood pressure were most effectively lowered by atenolol in accordance with the notion that enhanced SNS activity is an important mechanism behind the development and/or maintenance of hypertension in patients with OSA.

ACE inhibitors should not be viewed as having a primary therapy role in the patient with sleep apnea and hypertension, although the severity of the hypertension in the patient with sleep apnea and hypertension often requires that multiple antihypertensive drug classes (often including an ACE inhibitor or an ARB) be used if blood pressure is to be successfully lowered. In addition, ACE inhibitor and ARB therapy are therapeutic options in OSA patients because they can diminish the erythrocytosis (hypoxemia-related) often seen in these patients.

The use of an ACE inhibitor in the patient with OSA and hypertension should, however, occur cautiously because ACE inhibitors may also contribute to the severity of OSA, particularly in patients who develop cough and upper airway symptoms with their use. It has been suggested that patients with ACE inhibitor-related cough are more likely to exhibit rhinopharyngeal inflammation and, in turn, more readily collapse the upper airway. Cicolin et al reported a series of five ACE inhibitor-treated patients with cough whose AHI substantially improved upon ACE inhibitor discontinuation. In these patients, the improvement in the

AHI was associated with a decrease in exhaled NO—a presumed marker of airway inflammation. Accordingly, ACE inhibitors should be given cautiously (if at all) to patients with OSA and obvious upper airway inflammation. A therapeutic switch to an ARB in OSA patients with an ACE inhibitor-related cough also should be considered for the same reasons.

3. Do diuretics have a role in the treatment of OSA?

Diuretic therapy can have multiple roles in the patient with OSA and hypertension including facilitating blood-pressure reduction and/or decreasing extracellular fluid (ECF) volume, as well as serving as a respiratory stimulant. A diuretic is a useful adjunctive therapy for the typically complex hypertension observed in the patient with OSA. There is considerable heterogeneity among the available diuretics, with thiazide diuretic therapy most effectively reducing blood pressure. Loop diuretics are useful antihypertensive agents primarily when hypertension is being driven by significant ECF volume overload. The carbonic anhydrase inhibitor acetazolamide (Diamox®) is a mild diuretic whose benefit in OSA derives from its ability to cause a mild metabolic acidosis, and, in tandem with this, respiratory effort picks up and hypercapnia remits. In that regard, the nighttime administration of acetazolamide has been shown to decrease the frequency of obstructive events in patients with moderate-to-severe OSA.

Upper airway edema is a factor in pharyngeal collapsibility and likely contributes to the high prevalence of OSA in patients with heart disease. Bucca et al evaluated whether sleep-disordered breathing improved in patients with severe OSA and diastolic heart failure in response to intensive volume unloading with diuretics. Fifteen patients with severe OSA, hypertension, and diastolic heart failure received intravenous (IV) furosemide (Lasix®) (20 mg) and spironolactone (Aldactone®) (100 mg) twice daily for three consecutive days while hospitalized. Polysomnography (PSG) (assessment of the AHI), acoustic pharyngometry (determination of the oropharyngeal junction [OPJ] area), and functional lung parameters were measured before and after diuretic therapy.

Diuretic treatment resulted in a significant decrease in body weight, blood pressure, and AHI together with improvement in functional lung parameters and an increase in OPJ area. The decrease in AHI was significantly related to the amount of weight lost. These findings suggest that pharyngeal edema contributes to upper airway collapse during sleep, and are consistent with observations that neck circumference and pharyngeal size are influenced by changes in central blood pressure/volume. It remains to be determined whether long-term aggressive volume control in such patients will result in a more 'benign' course of progression for OSA.

4. What effect does CPAP have on blood pressure in the patient with OSA and hypertension?

CPAP, although the 'gold' standard treatment for OSA patients with moderate-to-severe disease, has an inconsistent effect on blood pressure in patients with OSA and hypertension. CPAP is delivered via a tightly fitting nasal mask, which in essence splints the pharyngeal airway during sleep so as to avoid collapse. CPAP is a cheap, noninvasive means of treating OSA, although it is poorly tolerated by many patients because of nasal congestion or the inability to maintain a tight fit of the mask to the face; accordingly, compliance can be quite variable with this therapy and may be one of the reasons that CPAP has such a variable effect on blood pressure. However, the technology of CPAP is rapidly evolving and increasingly offers a more customized therapy for delivery of positive airway pressure.

In patients with OSA, CPAP results in a marked reduction in sympathetic nerve traffic and, at the same time, checks the repetitive surges in blood pressure that occur at the end of an apneic episode. CPAP may offer its best benefit with those who have severe OSA because it is in these individuals that the greatest surges in blood pressure occur. CPAP can also be expected to induce a fall in the concentrations of several pressor and trophic substances that mark untreated OSA, which may have independent effects on both blood-pressure and cardiovascular outcomes.

Many studies show that CPAP reduces 24-hour ambulatory blood pressure, with greater treatment-related reductions in ambulatory mean blood-pressure (MBP) levels among patients with a more severe degree of OSA and a better daily dose of CPAP. The absolute blood-pressure drop that occurs with CPAP is particularly evident in those patients already receiving antihypertensive therapy and in those patients with faster heart rates. Seldom are the falls in blood pressure significant enough to allow for antihypertensive medication discontinuation or substantial reduction in medication doses; more often, CPAP facilitates the patient reaching his or her goal with existing therapies. These reductions in blood pressure are likely (but not proven) to contribute to a better prognosis in terms of adverse cardiovascular events.

5. *Do wakefulness-promoting agents, ie, modafinil (Provigil®), have a role in OSA-related hypertension?*

The treatment of OSA includes general noninvasive measures as well as selected therapies, including CPAP, surgery, and medication. Initial recommendations for all patients should include advice or therapy in how best to lose weight and avoiding the use of alcohol. If daytime somnolence and fatigue persist despite compliant use of CPAP or other oral appliances, therapy with pharmaceutical agents may prove beneficial. Excessive daytime somnolence typically has been addressed with stimulant-based therapies, ie, amphetamines, amphetamine derivatives (ie, methylphenidate [Concerta®, Daytrana™, Ritalin®]) However, because of the abuse potential for amphetamines, alternative therapies, ie, modafinil, have emerged as presumably safer alternatives.

The exact mechanism by which modafinil attenuates fatigue is incompletely understood. Unlike other central nervous system (CNS) agents that promote wakefulness but with the burden of a broad range of CNS stimulatory effects, modafinil has a selective effect on the hypothalamus and neither directly nor indirectly acts as a α_1-adrenergic agonist. The studies addressing the relationship between modafinil, blood pressure, and heart rate have produced conflicting results. Because the therapeutic gain for modafanil doses >200 mg/day is marginal, the fact that modafinil increases sympathetic activity, heart rate, and blood pressure at doses of ≥400 mg is of less concern possibly even with long-term use. Nonetheless, because patients with OSA typically have increased sympathetic nerve traffic and a baseline potential for cardiovascular complications, blood pressure and heart rate should be carefully monitored in OSA patients receiving modafinil.

6. Does aldosterone-receptor antagonist (ARA) therapy have a particular role in the patient with OSA and hypertension?

Obese hypertensive patients often have OSA, especially patients with excess fat deposits in their abdomen, which is often referred to as upper body obesity or visceral obesity. Obese hypertensives (with and without OSA) may have inappropriately raised levels of plasma aldosterone.

The mechanisms by which obesity and OSA increase aldosterone levels and raise blood pressure are incompletely understood; however, it has been suggested that SNS activation (common to OSA) and nonclassical adrenal stimuli, ie, oxidized products of linoleic acid (fatty tissue derived), promote release of this neurohormone.

There are two possible sequelae to explain excess circulating aldosterone concentrations in the patient with OSA. First, aldosterone can influence systemic blood pressure, and second, it can prompt sodium and water retention. The latter can result in extracellular fluid (ECF) volume expansion and fluid possibly shifting into interstitial compartments, ie, the soft tissue of the neck. If this occurs, airway resistance and/or an increased tendency for airway collapse may take place. These circumstances would seem to make an ARA, ie, spironolactone, a logical therapy choice; however, spironolactone has not been formally studied under these circumstances and its use remains empiric.

7. *Does proteinuria occur with OSA?*

OSA is significantly associated with increased urinary albumin excretion (UAE), especially among those with more severe disease, which may be a function of the generalized endothelial dysfunction that marks OSA. If present, low-level proteinuria in the OSA patient is related less to sleep apnea severity; rather, it is probably more closely tied to hypoxemia. Low-level proteinuria in the OSA patient does not seem to vary according to the sleep cycle. Clinically significant proteinuria is uncommon in stable patients with OSA. Accordingly, nephrotic-range proteinuria in patients with OSA should not be ascribed to sleep apnea and warrants a customary renal evaluation to exclude potentially treatable renal diseases. To date, the effect of CPAP on UAE has not been mechanistically evaluated; however, it would be reasonable to presume that an effective dose of CPAP would reduce UAE based on a number of its known positive effects, ie, blood-pressure reduction, improvement in endothelial function, decrease in oxidative stress, reduction in nocturnal hypoxemia/hypercarbia, a drop in inflammatory marker load.

Suggested Readings

Bucca CB, Brussino L, Battisti A, et al: Diuretics in obstructive sleep apnea with diastolic heart failure. *Chest* 2007;132:440-446.

Chrostowska M, Szczech R, Narkiewicz K: Antihypertensive therapy in the obese hypertensive patient. *Curr Opin Nephrol Hypertens* 2006;15:487-492.

Cicolin A, Mangiardi L, Mutani R, et al: Angiotensin-converting enzyme inhibitors and obstructive sleep apnea. *Mayo Clin Proc* 2006; 81:53-55.

Goncalves SC, Martinez D, Gus M, et al: Obstructive sleep apnea and resistant hypertension: a case-control study. *Chest* 2007;132:1858-1862.

Haentjens P, Van Meerhaeghe A, Moscariello A, et al: The impact of continuous positive airway pressure on blood pressure in patients with obstructive sleep apnea syndrome: evidence from a meta-analysis of placebo-controlled randomized trials. *Arch Intern Med* 2007;167:757-764.

Kuniyoshi FH, Somers VK: Sleep apnea in hypertension: when, how, and why should we treat? *Hypertension* 2006;47:818-819.

Mokhlesi B, Tulaimat A: Recent advances in obesity hypoventilation syndrome. *Chest* 2007;132:1322-1336.

Pratt-Ubunama MN, Nishizaka MK, Boedefeld RL, et al: Plasma aldosterone is related to severity of obstructive sleep apnea in subjects with resistant hypertension. *Chest* 2007;131:453-459.

Prisant LM, Dillard TA, Blanchard AR: Obstructive sleep apnea syndrome. *J Clin Hypertens (Greenwich)* 2006;8:746-750.

Rahmouni K, Correia ML, Haynes WG, et al: Obesity-associated hypertension: new insights into mechanisms. *Hypertension* 2005; 45:9-14.

Sim JJ, Rasgon SA, Derose SF: Sleep apnea and hypertension: prevalence in chronic kidney disease. *J Clin Hypertens (Greenwich)* 2007;9:837-841.

Chapter 4

Hypertension in Chronic Kidney Disease and Microalbuminuria

Chronic kidney disease (CKD) is defined as an estimated glomerular filtration rate (eGFR) <60 mL/min/1.73 m^2, or the presence of microalbuminuria or clinical proteinuria. The current hypertension guidelines suggest that the presence of either CKD or microalbuminuria should be considered a coronary artery disease (CAD) equivalent and that the recommended blood-pressure goal be set at <130/80 mm Hg.

Frequently Asked Questions

1. Why is evidence of CKD such a powerful marker for cardiovascular disease (CVD)?

Patients with CKD often have other established risk factors for CVD, ie, hypertension, dyslipidemia, diabetes. In addition, CKD patients may also have other nontraditional risk factors that could predispose them to CVD, ie, anemia, inflammation, disorders of calcium and phosphorous balance. The risk for CAD events is continuous and inversely proportional with estimated eGFR <60 mL/min and directly proportional with increasing levels of microalbuminuria or clinical proteinuria.

2. What is the optimal blood-pressure level in these high-risk patients?

Although treatment guidelines suggest that blood pressure <130/80 mm Hg is optimal, lower blood pressures may be beneficial, ie, blood-pressure levels necessary to normalize microalbuminuria or reduce clinical proteinuria by 50%. Since the glomerulus is a vascular structure, it is not surprising that blood-pressure levels affect its structure and function. Glomerular blood supply is optimal at a mean blood pressure approximately 50% to 75% of systemic blood pressure. Glomerular capillary pressure is tightly controlled via the autoregulatory relationships of the pre- and post-glomerular vascular beds. When the autoregulatory capability of the glomeruli is impaired through the development of blood-vessel disease, particularly the afferent arteriole, the glomeruli become more vulnerable to the effects of systemic blood pressure. As a result, the level of systemic blood pressure is often directly proportional to the progression rate of CKD, and the ambient level of albuminuria or proteinuria.

Numerous clinical studies in patients with nondiabetic or diabetic renal disease suggest that the optimal level of systolic blood pressure to prevent the progression of CKD is between 120 to 130 mm Hg. However, in some of these patients, lower blood-pressure goals may be preferable, perhaps as indicated by a concomitant reduction in urinary albumin excretion (UAE) or protein excretion. The clinical trial evidence suggests that those individuals whose microalbuminuria is normalized are less likely to progress to clinical proteinuria. In addition, those patients whose clinical proteinuria is reduced by at least 50% are less likely to progress to end-stage renal disease (ESRD). As a result, the reduction of proteinuria may serve as a biomeasure of an appropriate level of achieved blood pressure in a given patient. These observations may also explain why drugs that block the renin-angiotensin-aldosterone system (RAAS), ie, angiotensin-converting enzyme (ACE) inhibitors, angiotensin-receptor blockers (ARBs), or both, are a preferred therapeutic strategy as part of an effective blood-pressure-lowering regimen. Drugs that block the RAAS by antagonizing the effect of angiotensin II (Ang II) on the efferent glomerular arteriole are more effective in lowering glomerular capillary pressure as they lower systemic blood pressure than other commonly used antihypertensive drugs. However, it should be noted that patients with CKD require lower blood-pressure goals and also often require multiple antihypertensive drugs.

3. What is the optimal blood-pressure level for slowing the progression of CKD?

The majority of clinical trials in patients with CKD have evaluated the impact of different therapies on the progression rate of CKD compared with blood-pressure level. However, two important studies have looked at two levels of blood pressure that may affect the progression rate of CKD prospectively. The Modification of Diet in Renal Disease (MDRD) trial was primarily designed to evaluate the influence of dietary protein on the rate of CKD progression. However, the MDRD trial also assessed whether a blood-pressure level of 125/75 mm Hg was preferable to 140/90 mm Hg on the rate of lost kidney function over 3 years in patients with nondiabetic renal disease who had a eGFR between 13 and 55 mL/min. The results of this study indicate that the level of prestudy proteinuria influenced the rate of decline in kidney function and that the advantage of lower blood-pressure goals was most prominent in those with higher levels of pretreatment proteinuria. Those patients with >3 g of protein in urine/day demonstrated a statistically significant improvement in rate of loss of measured GFR, which was evident within 8 months of treatment. The MDRD trial also found that those patients with proteinuria levels between 1 and 3 g/24 hours did not benefit from the lower blood-pressure goals until after 24 months of therapy. Finally, those patients with <1 g of protein in urine/day did not benefit from the lower blood-pressure goal during the three years of the clinical trial. Thus, these results suggest that lower blood-pressure goals are most advantageous in patients with >1 g of protein in urine/day. However, the findings of the MDRD trial did not exclude the benefit of lower blood-pressure goals in patients with lesser degrees of proteinuria because these patients may require longer follow-up periods (ie, >3 years) to demonstrate the benefit of lower blood-pressure goals.

Similarly, the African-American Study of Kidney Disease (AASK) trial evaluated the same blood-pressure levels (ie, 140/90 mm Hg, 125/75 mm Hg) as the MDRD trial, as well as three different types of pharmacotherapy (ie, ACE inhibitor based, β-blocker based, calcium-channel blocker [CCB] based) in African Americans with either biopsy-proven or presumed hypertensive nephrosclerosis. Over the course of the 5-year trial, there was no evidence that showed a lower blood-pressure goal was advantageous on the rate of loss of measured GFR over time. However, the majority of patients had <1 g of protein in urine/day, which limited the power of the AASK trial to demonstrate the possible benefit of lower blood-pressure goals. Moreover, those patients with greater degrees of proteinuria (ie, >0.22 mg/g creatinine) did demonstrate a more substantial benefit of the ACE inhibitor-based regimen on the slope of loss of measured GFR during the clinical trial. Because this trial has been extended for another 5 years, more information will be available on whether or not lower blood-pressure goals and different types of pharmacotherapy will be advantageous in patients with lesser degrees of proteinuria and presumed hypertensive nephrosclerosis.

Secondary analysis of clinical trials in patients with nondiabetic renal disease suggests that lower achieved blood-pressure levels are important in delaying the progression of renal disease even after adjustment for the amount of proteinuria in urine. These studies also demonstrate the efficacy of RAAS blockers (eg, ACE inhibitors) along with lower blood-pressure goals in reducing the likelihood of doubling the serum-creatinine level, which can result in the development of ESRD. These studies also illustrate that systolic blood-pressure levels that approach 120 mm Hg may be optimal in the loss of measured GFR or eGFR over time.

Clinical studies in diabetics also illustrate the usefulness of lower blood-pressure goals in delaying the progression from microalbuminuria to clinical proteinuria, and from clinical proteinuria to ESRD. Patients with type 1 and type 2 diabetes with blood pressures in the 120 to 130 mm Hg range, if treated with a RAAS blocker (ie, an ACE inhibitor that is associated with a reduction in blood pressure), demonstrated an important and statistically significant reduction in risk in the progression from microalbuminuria to clinical proteinuria. This benefit was observed often within 2 years. What is not known from these studies is whether it is the effect of RAAS blockade, or lower blood pressure, or both, which results in the lesser likelihood in progression from microalbuminuria to macroalbuminuria. Interestingly, studies in patients with microalbuminuria and presumed normal blood pressure have been conducted. Yet, the achievement of lower blood pressure with RAAS blockade is associated with less likelihood of progression to proteinuria.

In diabetic patients with established nephropathy associated with reduced eGFR and clinical proteinuria, secondary analysis of the Irbesartan Type 2 Diabetic Nephropathy Trial (IDNT) and the Reduction of Endpoints in NIDDM with the Angiotensin II Antagonist Losartan (RENAAL) study clearly illustrates that renal disease progression is less common in those patients who achieve blood-pressure goals between 120 and 130 mm Hg as opposed to those who do not, regardless of the type of pharmacotherapy used to lower blood pressure.

In conclusion, the results of clinical trial data in patients with renal disease suggest that, whether patients are diabetic or not, blood-pressure goals between 120 and 130 mm Hg are optimal. The benefits of lower blood-pressure goals are more likely to be seen earlier in patients with more substantial degrees of proteinuria (>1 g/day). Longer duration of follow-up may be required to demonstrate the advantage of lower blood-pressure goals in the doubling of serum creatinine or reaching ESRD in patients with lesser degrees of proteinuria.

4. Is there a blood-pressure level that may be too low for the patient with renal disease?

There is substantial debate as to whether a J curve exists with regard to blood pressure and the progression rate of renal disease. This is an important consideration with regard to both renal disease progression as well as cardiovascular events.

The data with regard to renal disease progression is not well developed. Conceptually speaking, if a patient has or is at risk for ischemic nephropathy due to critical stenosis of the vascular supply to the kidneys, then there may be a finite level of blood pressure below which ischemic renal disease will progress. This may be associated with a loss of either measured GFR or eGFR over time as well as with shrinkage of kidney size as measured by ultrasound. However, the serum-creatinine level increases when lower blood pressure impairs renal perfusion, which should provide the clinician with the clue that evaluation of renal artery anatomy is required.

Because patients with renal disease are at an increased risk for CVD, concerns about reducing diastolic blood pressure below a certain threshold are of important concern. The secondary analysis of clinical trials that seek to lower blood pressure in patients with renal disease are often confounded by the different types of renal disease, the amount of proteinuria, and co-therapies for CVD. Despite this, there is the suggestion that, in nephropathic diabetics, systolic blood pressure in the 120 to 130 mm Hg range may be optimal, but that levels below that range (eg, <20 mm Hg) could be associated with an increased risk for cardiovascular events. However, lower blood pressure likely identifies patients with increased heart disease vs those receiving too much antihypertensive medication.

Heart rate may also be an important indicator of higher blood pressure and an increased risk of CKD. Because the majority of coronary artery hypertension occurs during diastole, the achieved heart rate with treatment may be a key consideration. Currently, it is safe to say that the achievement of a blood-pressure goal between 120 to 130 mm Hg may be considered optimal in the patient with CKD. More studies will be needed to evaluate the benefit vs risk ratio of blood-pressure goals <120 mm Hg in the patient with CKD.

5. Is there a difference between RAAS blockers and other antihypertensive medications in delaying the progression of renal disease?

In the aggregate, the majority of clinical trial data indicate that drugs that are effective in delaying the progression of renal disease must: (1) lower blood-pressure levels, preferably between 120 to 130 mm Hg and (2) block the RAAS. The data are consistent whether studying patients with diabetic or nondiabetic renal disease, particularly when there is >1 g of protein in urine/day. The latter factor is most important in interpreting the clinical trial data because, with lesser degrees of proteinuria, the duration of follow-up in the clinical trial may need to be extended to see the advantage of changes in blood-pressure goals and types of pharmacotherapies. In all major clinical trials of nondiabetic and diabetic renal disease with sufficient baseline proteinuria, and similar levels of treated blood pressure during follow-up, there is a uniformity in the results, which concluded that modifying the RAAS with either an ACE inhibitor or an ARB results in a reduction of renal end points. Invariably, this beneficial effect correlates with a reduction in proteinuria.

A few recently published meta-analyses have suggested that the only advantage of prescribing RAAS blockers is blood-pressure reduction, which can delay the progression of renal disease. However, these analyses are flawed because they have often combined clinical trials of patients with microalbuminuria and patients who have clinical proteinuria.

This limits the reliability of the analyses because a much longer follow-up period is required to evaluate renal events for those patients with a lesser degree of proteinuria.

6. *Is there a difference between an ACE inhibitor and an ARB on nephroprotection?*

There is only one head-to-head clinical trial that has been completed comparing an ACE inhibitor-based regimen with an ARB-based regimen in patients with diabetic nephropathy. The trial was small (n=136), but it lasted 5 years and did not show any difference in the risk of doubling of serum creatinine or of ESRD between the two treatment groups. As one looks at the clinical trial data in the aggregate, the majority of available data on kidney protection with ACE inhibitors is in patients with nondiabetic renal disease or in patients with type 1 diabetes and renal disease, whereas the data compiled on ARBs is largely derived from studies on renal disease associated with type 2 diabetes. Overall, there is uniformity in the benefits of using these drugs as part of an effective blood-pressure-lowering strategy that slows the progression of renal disease, whether a patient is diabetic or not.

7. *What are the best drugs to use with RAAS blockers to delay the progression of renal disease?*

This is a much more difficult question to answer because the majority of renal disease trials often prescribe multiple drugs to achieve necessary blood-pressure goals. It may be safer to say that drugs, such as diuretics or CCBs, which are known to work effectively with RAAS blockers, may be more useful. The key factor should always be to assist in the achievement of lower blood-pressure goals.

Some studies have suggested that nondihydropyridine CCBs (NCCBs) may be preferable to dihydropyridine CCBs (DCCBs) when used with RAAS blockers to reduce proteinuria. However, despite the fact that there is a difference in the antiproteinuric effects between DCCBs and NCCBs when used as a monotherapy, this does not appear to influence outcomes in proteinuric diabetics when they are also being treated with a RAAS blocker.

4

8. Is there an optimal dose of an ACE inhibitor or an ARB to delay the progression of renal disease?

Although many different types of ACE inhibitors and ARBs have been studied in patients with renal disease, most of the trials show that the highest approved dose for lowering blood pressure is the dose that reduces the risk of doubling serum creatinine or reaching ESRD. Thus, until we have more data using lower doses of these drugs, the full dose approved for blood pressure should be used based on the evidence from the clinical trials. Of course, adverse events, hypotension, and dosage adjustment based on the level of kidney function need to be considered.

9. Is it best to use an ACE inhibitor and an ARB together to provide protection against renal disease?

It is unknown whether one should use a full dose of an ACE inhibitor and an ARB together as part of an effective blood-pressure-lowering regimen to slow the rate of progression of renal disease. Although some smaller studies have demonstrated that this approach may be more effective in reducing microalbuminuria or clinical proteinuria, it is not known whether this will translate into fewer renal disease events. One small study from Japan in patients with nondiabetic glomerulonephritis and clinical proteinuria suggested that using a full dose of an ARB and an ACE inhibitor may be preferable to using a full dose of an ACE inhibitor or an ARB alone in reducing proteinuria and changing the eGFR over time. However, these results should be viewed with caution because they were derived from a small study population. This study's results need to be reproduced in a large-scale study of patients with nondiabetic and diabetic renal disease.

10. Is reduction of proteinuria or microalbuminuria the best measure of therapeutic success of a given regimen in delaying the progression of renal disease?

Renal disease progression is a heterogeneous process. It is likely that blood-pressure level may be the critical factor in the progression of renal disease. The transglomerular passage of albumin and reuptake process through the renal tubular epithelia may result in an inflammatory process in the kidneys that ultimately leads to the progression of renal disease. Whether it is the blood-pressure reduction that results in less hydraulic pressure and less filtration of proteins or it is the specific antiproteinuric properties, ie, RAAS blockers, which reduce the progression rate of renal disease is unknown. However, the results of clinical trials do suggest that the reduction of microalbuminuria is associated with less progression to clinical proteinuria and the reduction of clinical proteinuria is associated with less risk of doubling serum creatinine or reaching ESRD. These observations are more often associated with lower levels of achieved blood pressure, but not uniformly. Blood-pressure treatment goals that optimally reduce proteinuria may serve as a more accurate biomeasure for optimal treatment levels of blood pressure in an individual patient. More studies will need to be completed to evaluate the clinical relevance of proteinuria reduction as a measure of therapeutic success in the patient with nondiabetic or diabetic renal disease.

Suggested Readings

Agodoa LY, Appel L, Bakris GL, et al: Effect of ramipril vs amlodipine on renal outcomes in hypertensive nephrosclerosis: a randomized controlled trial. *JAMA* 2001;285:2719-2728.

Bakris GL, Weir MR, Secic M, et al: Differential effects of calcium antagonist subclasses on markers of nephropathy progression. *Kidney Int* 2004;65:1991-2002.

Bakris GL, Williams M, Dworkin L, et al: Preserving renal function in adults with hypertension and diabetes: a consensus approach.

National Kidney Foundation Hypertension and Diabetes Executive Committees Working Group. *Am J Kidney Dis* 2000;36:646-661.

Barnett AH, Bain SC, Bouter P, et al: Angiotensin-receptor blockade versus converting-enzyme inhibition in type 2 diabetes and nephropathy. *N Engl J Med* 2004;35:1952-1961.

Chobanian AV, Bakris GL, Black HR, et al: The Seventh Report of the Joint National Committee on Prevention, Detection, Evaluation, and Treatment of High Blood Pressure: the JNC 7 report. *JAMA* 2003; 289:2560-2572.

Hilgers KF, Mann JF: ACE inhibitors versus AT(1) receptor antagonists in patients with chronic renal disease. *J Am Soc Nephrol* 2002;13:1100-1108.

Jafar TH, Stark PC, Schmid CH, et al, and the AIPRD Study Group: Progression of chronic kidney disease: the role of blood pressure control, proteinuria, and angiotensin-converting enzyme inhibition; a patient-level meta-analysis. *Ann Intern Med* 2003;139:244-252.

Klahr S, Levey AS, Beck GJ, et al: The effects of dietary protein restriction and blood-pressure control on the progression of chronic renal disease. Modification of Diet in Renal Disease Study Group. *N Engl J Med* 1994;330:877-884.

Nakao N, Yoshimura A, Morita H, et al: Combination treatment of angiotensin-II receptor blocker and angiotensin-converting-enzyme inhibitor in non-diabetic renal disease (COOPERATE): a randomised controlled trial. *Lancet* 2003;361:117-124.

Pohl MA, Blumenthal S, Cordonnier DJ, et al: Independent and additive impact of blood pressure control and angiotensin II receptor blockade on renal outcomes in the irbesartan diabetic nephropathy trial: clinical implications and limitations. *J Am Soc Nephrol* 2005; 16:3027-3037.

Sarnak MJ, Levey AS, Schoolwerth AC, et al: Kidney disease as a risk factor for development of cardiovascular disease: a statement from the American Heart Association Councils on Kidney in Cardiovascular Disease, High Blood Pressure Research, Clinical Cardiology, and Epidemiology and Prevention. *Circulation* 2003;108:2154-2169.

Weir MR: Microalbuminuria and cardiovascular disease. *Clin J Am Soc Nephrol* 2007;2:581-590.

Chapter 5

Diuretics

Diuretics are tools of considerable therapeutic importance. First, diuretics effectively reduce blood pressure, while simultaneously decreasing the morbidity and mortality from hypertension. Diuretics are currently recommended by the Joint National Commission on Prevention, Detection, Evaluation, and Treatment of High Blood Pressure (JNC 7) as a first-line therapy for hypertension. In addition, diuretics continue to be an important component of heart failure therapy because they improve the symptoms of congestion, which epitomize the more advanced stages of heart failure.

The exact means by which a thiazide diuretic lowers blood pressure is unclear. The effect of a thiazide diuretic on blood pressure may be separated into three seemingly sequential response phases: acute, subacute, and chronic, which correspond to periods of more or less 1 to 2 weeks, several weeks, and several months, respectively. In the acute response phase, the blood-pressure-lowering effect of a diuretic is coupled to a reduction in extracellular fluid (ECF) volume (<12%) and a corresponding fall in cardiac output. The early response (ie, first 2 to 4 days of treatment) to a thiazide diuretic, in the setting of a no-salt-added diet (100 to 150 mmol/day), results in a net sodium loss of 100 to 300 mmol, which translates into a 1 to 2 L decrease in ECF volume. This decrease in plasma volume diminishes venous return and drops cardiac output, establishing the basis for the initial blood-pressure fall with a thiazide diuretic. The change in plasma volume also can stimulate the sympathetic nervous system (SNS) and the renin-angiotensin-aldosterone system (RAAS), which govern the acute decrease in blood pressure. In due course, thiazide diuretic effects on plasma volume and cardiac output lessen in importance, although blood pressure remains lowered. During the subacute response phase of the treatment response (ie, first few weeks), plasma volume returns to slightly less than pretreatment levels despite the continued administration of a diuretic. The subacute response phase with thiazide diuretics is a transition period during which both plasma volume and resistance factors contribute to the reduction in blood pressure.

In the chronic response phase of therapy, the vasodepressor influence of a diuretic develops into a process mechanistically driven by a reduction in total peripheral resistance (TPR). There is no simple explanation for the drop in TPR that accompanies long-term diuretic use. The decrease in TPR during prolonged therapy has been attributed to several factors—changes in the ionic content of vascular smooth muscle cells, altered ion gradients across smooth muscle cells and/or potassium-channel activation, and changes in membrane-bound blood-pressure activity. The ability of thiazide diuretics to reduce blood pressure may be critically linked to the presence of functioning renal tissue, thus, these drugs do not reduce ATPase in functionally anuric patients undergoing maintenance hemodialysis. Whatever the mechanism of thiazide-related blood-pressure reduction, it can be long lasting because a residual blood-pressure reduction can be seen several weeks after the withdrawal of thiazide diuretics (even without interposing nonpharmacologic treatments for the maintenance of blood-pressure control). However, the residual blood-pressure-lowering effect of thiazide diuretics has not been carefully compared with the blood-pressure-lowering effects of nondiuretic antihypertensive medication drug classes.

Frequently Asked Questions

1. How are diuretic-related side effects categorized?

Diuretic-related side effects can be separated into several categories including those with known mechanisms, ie, electrolyte defects and/or metabolic abnormalities, and those that are less well understood mechanistically, ie, impotence and those side effects that are perceived to be idiosyncratic. In addition, various drug/drug interactions can occur with diuretics. Diuretic-related side effects are more common and often are of greater intensity with loop diuretics. Electrolyte side effects are more common with longer acting thiazide compounds, ie, chlorthalidone (Thalitone®), metolazone (Zaroxolyn®). Among the thiazide diuretics, indapamide (Lozol®) has been touted as distinctive because it does not cause significant metabolic derangements. However, when given in equivalent doses to hydrochlorothiazide (Esidrix®, Microzide®), there is little that separates hydrochlorothiazide and indapamide with regard to side effects.

Idiosyncratic side effects relating to diuretic therapy can derive from allergic/immunologic reactions and/or a toxic response to metabolites. The circumstance under which allergic or idiosyncratic (the terms 'allergic' and 'idiosyncratic' are often used interchangeably) reactions is most clinically relevant is when an allergy exists to a sulfonamide antibiotic, and a decision has to be made as to whether a sulfonamide nonantibiotic (ie, a diuretic) can be safely given. Patients with a history of hypersensitivity to sulfonamide antibiotics are at even greater risk for ensuing reactions to penicillins than they are to sulfonamide diuretics. Prescribers should appreciate that patients with a history of allergic reactions to sulfonamide antibiotic drugs may be at increased risk for all drug-induced adverse events of a seemingly allergic nature.

2. Does the development of hyponatremia after being prescribed a diuretic always require that the diuretic be discontinued?

Hyponatremia is an uncommon, but serious, complication of diuretic therapy. Thiazide diuretics are more likely to cause hyponatremia than loop diuretics. Loop diuretics inhibit sodium transport in the renal medulla and prevent the generation of a maximal osmotic gradient, thus, urinary concentrating ability is impaired with loop diuretics. Alternatively, thiazide diuretics increase sodium excretion and preclude maximal urine dilution, while maintaining the concentrating capacity of the kidneys. When diuretic-related hyponatremia occurs, it is typically in elderly females and is usually seen within the first 2 weeks of therapy; however, diuretic-related hyponatremia can occur even after several years of therapy. Multiple factors contribute to females developing diuretic-related hyponatremia including age, a reduced body mass, an exaggerated natriuretic response to a thiazide diuretic, a diminished capacity to excrete free water, and what is usually a self-imposed low solute intake. Independent of these risk factors, it has been suggested that the preponderance of thiazide-induced hyponatremia in females is related to thiazide diuretics being more frequently prescribed for women.

Mild, asymptomatic, diuretic-related hyponatremia (ie, typically between 130 to 135 mmol/L) does not require that the diuretic be discontinued, if it is determined to be a nonprogressive form of hyponatremia. A reduction in fluid intake and/or a modest increase in solute intake as well as a reduction in diuretic dose are usually sufficient to manage serum sodium in the 130 to 135 mmol/L range. Serum-sodium values <130 mmol/L require more intense medical management as well as an immediate discontinuation of the diuretic. Although diuretic therapy can be tried again in such patients, in most instances, the hyponatremia recurs rather quickly.

3. *Are there differences in the various thiazide diuretics, or is there a class effect for all thiazide drugs?*

The concept of a class effect has been applied to both loop and thiazide diuretics in the management of hypertension. The idea of a class effect for thiazide diuretics is one disseminated by many clinicians, but it has little experimental support. Much of the recent debate on a thiazide diuretic class effect has centered on the similarities (or not) between chlorthalidone and hydrochlorothiazide. The concept of a class effect with thiazide diuretics needs to be thought of in two ways: first, blood pressure lowering, and, second, cardiovascular event-rate reduction. Chlorthalidone and hydrochlorothiazide are fundamentally different diuretics in that chlorthalidone has a considerably longer duration of diuretic action and is a more effective antihypertensive compound than hydrochlorothiazide. Studies by Ernst et al argue convincingly that blood pressure is reduced more effectively with chlorthalidone than with hydrochlorothiazide at a fixed-dose ratio of 2:1 (hydrochlorothiazide 50 mg: chlorthalidone 25 mg). This blood-pressure difference, as determined by ambulatory blood-pressure monitoring, was particularly impressive in the evening hours. The reduction in systolic blood pressure during nighttime hours was -13.5 ± 1.9 mm Hg for chlorthalidone vs -6.4 ± 1.7 mm Hg for hydrochlorothiazide, which was highly significant. Chlorthalidone has also had a more consistent pattern of favorable outcomes than hydrochlorothiazide. If for no other reason than more effective blood-pressure reduction, chlorthalidone should be used with more regularity especially in the difficult-to-treat patient with resistant hypertension.

4. *Do lower diuretic doses decrease the likelihood of side effects?*

In the early days of diuretic use, doses were unnecessarily high because it was believed that 'if a little is good, more is better'; however, it was soon recognized that the dose/blood-pressure response for a thiazide diuretic (ie, hydrochlorothiazide) was relatively flat beyond a daily dose of 25 mg, and much of the negative metabolic experience with diuretics occurred at the very-high-dosage levels (ie, 100 to 200 mg/day). It is clear that lower doses of thiazide diuretics significantly reduce the risk of developing hypokalemia, hyperglycemia, hyperlipidemia, and/or hyperuricemia. As a result, dosing >25 mg is not routinely recommended. While higher doses can lead to some modest further reductions in blood pressure and thereby increase blood-pressure control rates, the risk of biochemical abnormalities is greatly increased and there appears to be less of a reduction in the anticipated cardiovascular risk.

5. Are there clinically relevant changes in lipid levels with diuretics?

Diuretics increase total serum cholesterol, low-density lipoprotein cholesterol (LDL-C), and triglycerides (Tgs), and they may slightly reduce high-density lipoprotein cholesterol (HDL-C). These effects occur with both thiazide and loop diuretics. Among thiazide diuretics, indapamide may influence lipid levels less; however, this may be a function of dose selection when indapamide is compared with other thiazide-like compounds. The potassium-sparing diuretic spironolactone (Aldactone®) is neutral with regard to lipid changes. The effects of diuretics on lipids may be more pronounced in males, blacks, diabetics, and nonresponders to diuretic treatment. The mechanism for this effect is not clear, but it may be related to higher insulin levels, hypomagnesemia, or reflex activation of the RAAS and SNS as a consequence of plasma-volume depletion. Large studies have found that these effects on lipid parameters wane over time and changes in lipid parameters are often no different than what are seen with other antihypertensive agents, ie, angiotensin-converting enzyme (ACE) inhibitors, calcium-channel blockers (CCBs). While it is not clear whether the effect of diuretics on lipids is dose related, studies that have used low diuretic doses have generally found a less negative effect on lipid parameters. In addition, any negative effects on lipids that occur with diuretics may be lessened by co-administration of an ACE inhibitor.

6. How are acid base changes associated with an optimally managed diuretic?

Mild diuretic-induced metabolic alkalosis is a common feature of thiazide diuretic therapy, particularly at higher doses. Severe metabolic alkalosis is much less frequent, and when it occurs, it is typically in association with high-dose loop diuretic therapy. The development of severe metabolic alkalosis can lead to hypoventilation and the establishment of a mixed acid-base disorder that may make weaning the ventilated patient a more complicated process. The generation of a metabolic alkalosis with diuretic therapy is primarily due to contraction of the ECF space caused by urinary losses of a relatively bicarbonate (HCO_3-) free fluid. Diuretic-induced metabolic alkalosis is best managed through the administration of potassium and/or sodium chloride, although sodium chloride administration may be impractical in already volume-expanded patients (ie, heart failure patients). In such cases, a potassium-sparing diuretic or a carbonic anhydrase inhibitor, ie, acetazolamide, may be considered. Metabolic alkalosis impairs the natriuretic response to loop diuretics and may play a role in the diuretic resistance sometimes found in the heart failure patient. All potassium-sparing diuretics can cause hyperkalemic metabolic acidosis, which in elderly patients, or in those with renal impairment or heart failure, can reach life-threatening levels.

7. How often does impotence occur with diuretic therapy?

The adverse effects of thiazide and thiazide-like diuretics on male sexual function, including decreased libido, erectile dysfunction, and difficulty ejaculating, have been reported with an incidence range from 3% to 32%. As an example, in the Medical Research Council (MRC) trial in which 15,000 hypertensive subjects received either placebo, a thiazide (bendrofluazide), or a β-blocker (propranolol [Inderal®]) for 5 years, impotence was 22-fold and 4-fold higher with bendrofluazide compared with placebo or β-blocker, respectively. The mechanism through which thiazides affect erectile function or libido is unclear. Low serum potassium or a drop in blood pressure do not seem to correlate with the sexual side effects of a diuretic. It has been suggested that thiazides have a direct effect on vascular smooth muscle cells and/or decrease the responsiveness to catecholamines; however, patients with diuretic-related impotence respond to sildenafil (Revatio™, Viagra®) and do so without any additional drop in blood pressure.

Impotence and decreased libido are the more frequent sexual side effects with spironolactone. Gynecomastia, another frequent complication of spironolactone therapy, may be coupled with mastodynia and is typically bilateral. One study of 699 men reported that 13% (19/699) of men prescribed spironolactone alone or with another antihypertensive treatment developed dose-related gynecomastia, which was reversible. The sexual side effects of spironolactone have been attributed to endocrine dysfunction because spironolactone is structurally similar to sex hormones and inhibits the binding of dihydrotestosterone (DHT) to androgen receptors, thus increasing testosterone clearance. Eplerenone is a more selective aldosterone- receptor antagonist (ARA) and does not have the sexual side effects observed with spironolactone.

8. What is the best way to manage hyperuricemia in a patient with gout and hypertension when diuretic therapy is necessary?

Thiazide diuretics therapy increases serum-urate concentrations by as much as 35%, an effect related to decreased renal clearance of urate, which is most prominent in those with the highest pretherapy urate clearance values. Decreased urate clearance may be linked to increased reabsorption secondary to diuretic-related ECF volume depletion and/or competition for tubular secretion because thiazide diuretics and urate undergo tubular secretion by the same organic anion transporter pathway. Diuretic-related hyperuricemia is dose dependent and is important for two reasons—as a precipitant of gout and as it relates to its potential effect on cardiovascular event rates.

Diuretic-related hyperuricemia does not typically precipitate a gouty attack, unless the patient has an underlying gouty tendency or serum-urate concentrations routinely >12 mg/dL. In the MRC trial, patients receiving high-dose thiazide diuretics had significantly more withdrawals for gout than did placebo-treated patients (4.4 vs 0.1/1,000 patient-years). In the Systolic Hypertension in the Elderly Program (SHEP) trial, those patients with a serum-uric acid increase ≥0.06 mmol/L (median change) in the active treatment group had the same risk of coronary events as the placebo group. This observation suggests that diuretic-related hyperuricemia offsets the positive cardiovascular benefits of the blood-pressure reduction achieved through diuretic therapy.

Allopurinol (Aloprim™, Lopurin®, Zyloprim®) should not be routinely started for asymptomatic diuretic-related hyperuricemia. If a gouty attack occurs in a diuretic-treated patient, the diuretic in use should be temporarily discontinued and some consideration given to starting allopurinol once the gouty attack has quieted and prior to restarting the diuretic. In so doing, a diuretic can often be restarted at a lower, but still effective dose; however, in the process, careful attention should be paid to avoid excessive volume contraction. Allopurinol is a renally cleared compound, and it should be used cautiously (dose adjusted according to the level of renal function) in patients receiving a thiazide diuretic because allopurinol hypersensitivity reactions are more common with this combination. A final consideration is what steps to take in a patient with diuretic-related hyperuricemia who is intolerant of allopurinol. One option to consider is allopurinol desensitization. However, this is a cumbersome process. A more ready alternative is the use of the angiotensin-receptor blocker (ARB) losartan (Cozaar®), which is a uricosuric compound. Losartan can be safely given with a reduction of 1 mg/dL in serum-uric acid on average with no risk of acute urate nephropathy and/or uric acid stones.

9. How is diuretic-related hypokalemia most effectively managed?

The lowest rates of cardiovascular risk and glucose intolerance appear to occur at serum-potassium values between 4 to 4.5 mmol/L; thus, a serum-potassium level in this range is typically targeted in the diuretic-treated patient. Not allowing hypokalemia to occur in the first place is a preferred strategy in the diuretic-treated patient. This is best accomplished with the use of the lowest diuretic dose possible accompanied by a reduction in dietary sodium intake. Potassium supplements are the next choice, and potassium chloride is the best potassium salt to use because its use also facilitates correction of the mild metabolic alkalosis seen in diuretic-treated patients.

Potassium-sparing diuretics (ie, amiloride, triamterene [Dyrenium®]) and ARAs (ie, eplerenone [Inspra®], spironolactone) are probably better choices than potassium supplements in preventing or treating hypokalemia. Potassium supplements can normalize serum-potassium values in the hypokalemic patient, but they do little to correct the accompanying cellular deficiency of potassium. Potassium-sparing diuretics increase serum-potassium values and restore the cellular complement of potassium in the hypokalemic patient. However, this effect is extremely dose dependent, and, therefore, poorly predictable, with patients becoming normokalemic, remaining hypokalemic, or possibly developing hyperkalemia. As a matter of reference, in a study that examined the effect of various treatments on hypokalemia (range=3.28 to 3.68 mmol/L), it was observed that the potassium supplements amiloride, spironolactone, and triamterene increased serum potassium by 0.32, 0.39, 0.46, and 0.65 mmol/L, respectively.

The patient prone to the development of hyperkalemia with a potassium-sparing diuretic usually is one with more significant renal insufficiency and/or concomitantly receiving potassium supplements, patients taking low-salt and no-salt dietary products (60 mmol/tsp), and/or those receiving an ACE inhibitor or an ARB. While these therapies can be used together in most patients, the increased monitoring of electrolytes is necessary for those patients with a reduced glomerular filtration rate (GFR) (ie, chronic kidney disease [CKD]), individuals who develop acute or chronic renal failure, metabolic acidosis, hyporeninemic hypoaldosteronism, and those receiving heparin therapy (including subcutaneous heparin regimens) and nonsteroidal anti-inflammatory drugs (NSAIDs), including over-the-counter (OTC) preparations.

10. Is the change in glucose concentration experienced with a diuretic important?

Prolonged thiazide diuretic therapy can lead to glucose intolerance and may occasionally precipitate type 2 diabetes. Short-term metabolic studies, epidemiologic studies, and a variety of clinical trials suggest a connection between ongoing thiazide diuretic use and the onset of type 2 diabetes. However, it should be noted that interpretation of these studies is confounded by multiple factors including differing definitions of new-onset diabetes, small numbers of patients in the studies, inadequate comparison groups, relatively limited periods of follow-up, selection criteria that limit the generalization of the findings, and study designs that prohibited valid comparisons among antihypertensive drug classes. Diuretic-associated glucose intolerance appears to be dose related, less common with loop diuretics, not present with spironolactone, and reversible upon withdrawal of the agent, although the data on reversibility in hydrochlorothiazide-treated patients is somewhat conflicting. Other drug classes, ie, ACE inhibitors, ARBs, are associated with less incidence of new-onset diabetes The extent to which either of these drug classes reduces the diabetogenic potential of thiazide diuretics remains to be determined.

Hyperglycemia has been seen as both a cause and an effect of hypokalemia. A recent meta-analysis of 59 studies involving 83 thiazide diuretic treatment arms found a significant correlation between the degree of hypokalemia and the increase in plasma glucose. There was also evidence that prevention of hypokalemia with potassium supplementation lessened the degree to which plasma glucose increases. Potassium deficiency inhibits insulin secretion from pancreatic β-cells, which is one of several possible mechanisms that explains how hypokalemia modifies glucose homeostasis. One reason why ACE inhibitors and ARBs may reduce glucose intolerance and new-onset diabetes is that both drug classes can modestly increase serum-potassium values. While not as extensively studied, magnesium deficiency, which is often accompanied by hypokalemia, is also associated with glucose intolerance.

Suggested Readings

Carter BL, Sica DA: Strategies to improve the cardiovascular risk profile of thiazide-type diuretics as used in the management of hypertension. *Expert Opin Drug Saf* 2007;6:583-594.

Ernst ME, Carter BL, Goerdt CJ, et al: Comparative antihypertensive effects of hydrochlorothiazide and chlorthalidone on ambulatory and office blood pressure. *Hypertension* 2006;47:352-358.

Fogari R, Zoppi A: Effects of antihypertensive therapy on sexual activity in hypertensive men. *Curr Hypertens Rep* 2002;4:202-210.

Johnson BF, Saunders R, Hickler R, et al: The effects of thiazide diuretics upon plasma lipoproteins. *J Hypertens* 1986;4:235-239.

Neutel JM, Black HR, Weber MA: Combination therapy with diuretics: an evolution of understanding. *Am J Med* 1996;101(3A):61S-70S.

Psaty B, Smith N, Siscovick D, et al: Health outcomes associated with antihypertensive therapies used as first-line agents: A systematic review and meta-analysis. *JAMA* 1997;277:739-745.

Reyes AJ: Cardiovascular drugs and serum uric acid. *Cardiovasc Drugs Ther* 2003;17:397-414.

Sica DA: Diuretic-related side effects: development and treatment. *J Clin Hypertens (Greenwich)* 2004;6:532-540.

Strom BL, Schinnar R, Apter AJ, et al: Absence of cross-reactivity between sulfonamide antibiotics and sulfonamide nonantibiotics. *N Engl J Med* 2003;349:1628-1635.

Zillich AJ, Garg J, Basu S, et al: Thiazide diuretics, potassium, and the development of diabetes: a quantitative review. *Hypertension* 2006;48:219-224.

Chapter 6

β-Blockade

β-Blockers have been available for more than three decades. There are numerous β-blockers, each presumably distinctive, one from the other. The various β-blockers can be conveniently classified by their relative selectivity for the β_1 receptor (primarily in the heart) and the presence and/or absence of intrinsic sympathomimetic activity (ISA). Although there are clear pharmacologic differences among the drugs in this class, in general, such dissimilarities are of limited clinical significance relative to blood-pressure control.

The therapeutic efficacy and safety of β-adrenergic-blocking drugs has been well established after 40 years of continuous use. Their clinical utility has also been confirmed in patients with angina pectoris, cardiac arrhythmias, heart failure, and hypertension, and for reducing the risk of mortality and possibly nonfatal reinfarction in survivors of acute myocardial infarction (MI). These drugs may also be of use in reducing cardiovascular morbidity and mortality in hypertensive patients.

The competitive inhibition of β-adrenergic activity by β-blockers produces numerous functional effects with the potential to regulate blood pressure including a reduction in cardiac output, a fall in renin release, perhaps a decrease in sympathetic outflow, and a presynaptic blockade, which inhibits catecholamine release. The effect of β-blockers on peripheral vascular resistance is still argued, although a small decrease in resistance usually follows from chronic β-blocker administration. However, the exact way in which β-blockers reduce blood pressure remains unclear, and it is likely that their mechanism of action differs among patients.

There is no real predictor of response to monotherapy with a β-blocker. Alternatively, there are patient characteristics that predict a poor responder status, including being black and advancing age. β-Blockers given with a diuretic or a dihydropyridine calcium-channel blocker (DCCB), either as fixed-dose or individual monotherapies, significantly reduce blood pressure. The physiologic rationale supporting either of these combinations is understandable. β-Blockers will blunt the renin-angiotensin-aldosterone system (RAAS) activation brought on by diuretic therapy, while the diuretic component of the combination curbs any sodium retention provoked by β-blockers. This is particularly true when diuretic or β-blocker doses are high. Alternatively, when a β-blocker is given with a DCCB, any rise in heart rate that occurs with the latter can be lessened. There is little incremental benefit when a β-blocker is added to either an angiotensin-converting enzyme (ACE) inhibitor or an angiotensin-receptor blocker (ARB).

Most β-blockers, at least in the usual dose range, should not be used in patients with asthma, acutely decompensated heart failure, heart block (greater than first degree), or sick sinus syndrome. These drugs should also be used with caution in insulin-dependent diabetes because they can worsen glycemic control, mask the adrenergically driven symptoms of hypoglycemia, prolong recovery from hypoglycemia, or increase the magnitude of the pressor response to hypoglycemia. β-Blockers should also not be stopped suddenly in patients with active ischemic heart disease. Finally, β-blockers can worsen claudication and Raynaud's phenomenon.

Frequently Asked Questions

1. Should β-blockers be used routinely as first-line therapy in the treatment of hypertension?

For more than three decades, β-blockers have been commonly used in the treatment of hypertension, and, until recently, national and international guidelines still recommended these compounds as first-line agents. However, recent meta-analyses and systematic reviews indicate that, in patients with uncomplicated hypertension (compared with other antihypertensive agents), first-line therapy with β-blockers is associated with an increased risk of stroke (especially in the elderly) with no benefit for end points, ie, all-cause mortality, cardiovascular morbidity and mortality.

As a point of comparison, diuretic therapy has consistently been proven superior to β-blockers with regard to numerous outcomes including fatal and nonfatal strokes, cardiovascular events, and all-cause mortality. Moreover, most of the beneficial effects and nonharmful effects of β-blockers in the major clinical trials appear to be the result of add-on diuretic therapy. The inability of β-blockers to offer cardiovascular benefits in the uncomplicated patient with hypertension may in large measure relate to the β-blocker that was used in most of the trials (ie, atenolol [Tenormin®]), which is a generally weaker blood-pressure-lowering compound that also has little discernable effect on central aortic pressures.

Given the increased risk of stroke, a failure to lower central aortic pressures, the minimal effect on regression of left-ventricular hypertrophy (LVH) and/or improvement of endothelial dysfunction, and frequent adverse side effects, the risk/benefit ratio for β-blockers is unacceptable for use as first-line therapy in the uncomplicated hypertensive patient. These findings related to the use of β-blockers have begun to be seriously considered by guideline committees. For example, a joint initiative between the National

Institute for Health and Clinical Excellence (NICE) and the British Hypertension Society (BHS) has recommended that, in the uncomplicated hypertensive patient, β-blockers no longer be considered as suitable options for first-line therapy. However, the NICE guidelines do not offer a blanket censure of β-blocker use because they remain efficacious agents for the treatment of heart failure, certain arrhythmias, hypertrophic obstructive cardiomyopathy, and in patients with a previous MI.

2. *What patient populations are typically most responsive to β-blocker therapy?*

Hypertension—β-Blockers have been proposed as effective monotherapy agents for young to middle-aged hypertensives, especially white males, and in patients with myocardial ischemia, hypertrophic obstructive cardiomyopathy, a hyperdynamic circulation, high levels of anxiety and/or stress, and essential tremor and/or headaches. β-Blockers have also proven useful in treating perioperative hypertension. Alternatively, it has been suggested that the response to β-blockers is less so in patients who tend to have lower levels of plasma-renin activity (PRA), ie, blacks and the elderly. The evidence supporting a lesser response for blacks is persuasive and consistent. The issue of β-blocker response in the elderly strongly supports the belief that the elderly are less responsive to these medications. β-Blockers however, can be used to good effect when the elderly have comorbid conditions, ie, coronary artery disease (CAD) or essential tremor.

An additional consideration in assessing the effects of β-blockers is their inherent dose-response relationship. Most β-blockers have a flat dose-response curve, as has been repeatedly shown with atenolol (Tenormin®) and propranolol (Inderal®). For example, atenolol given at a dose of 25 mg/day has been shown to be as effective as doses of 50, 75, or 100 mg/day. In addition, in certain instances, upward dose titration of a β-blocker results in loss of previously established blood-pressure control when the increase causes salt and water retention and plasma-volume expansion. Alternatively, in pulse-rate-driven forms of hypertension, dose escalation can provide additional benefits if the pulse rate can be further reduced.

Elevated Heart Rate—In recent years, considerable evidence has been assembled in support of the theory that resting heart rate is a major correlate of blood pressure, that it may herald the development of sustained hypertension in subjects with normal or borderline hypertension values, and that it is associated with a heightened risk of both cardiovascular and noncardiovascular death. Despite the inherent difficulties in interpreting resting clinic heart rate, in most instances it has proven predictive of the future development of hypertension particularly with resting heart rates >80 beats/minute. High heart rates, in otherwise healthy individuals, reflect an imbalance of autonomic function marked by either increased sympathetic activity and/or reduced vagal activity. In the hypertensive patient, heightened sympathetic activity is coupled to a number of other cardiovascular risk factors, including insulin resistance/dyslipidemia, increased hematocrit, and the development of LVH. Furthermore, the hemodynamic consequences of an increased pulse rate, ie, increased shear forces, independently damage the vascular endothelium, and thereby facilitate the development of atherosclerosis. An augmentation of shear forces is importantly linked to the rate-pressure product, among other permissive variables.

As is the case in the treatment of hypertension, nonpharmacologic measures are an important element of treating the patient with an elevated heart rate. Such measures include reduction in caloric intake, restricting the intake of alcohol and caffeinated beverages, potentially increasing sodium intake (if sodium intake is low on a self-imposed basis), and embarking on a program of regular physical exercise. In particular, physical exercise (as conditioning improves) may effectively reduce resting heart rate. In assessing heart-rate response to nonpharmacologic measures (as is the case for baseline heart rates), there should be some standardization to the process related to observer, body position, environmental factors, and psychic stimuli. Heart rate should also preferentially be assessed in an out-of-office setting to eliminate the in-office confounding effect of the alerting reaction on heart rate.

Although there is no published evidence to demonstrate that cardiac slowing is beneficial in the patient with hypertension and an elevated heart rate (ie, >80 beats/minute), it would appear that β-blocker therapy (or, if contraindicated, rate-lowering CCB therapy) is indicated in such patients; however, there is no definitive evidence available that might guide therapeutic efforts as to what degree heart rate should be reduced. However, epidemiologic data have demonstrated that a 10% to 12% reduction in heart rate is associated with a 20% to 40% reduction in cardiovascular morbidity and mortality.

Mid-to-high range doses of a β-blocker can be expected to reduce heart rate by 10% to 12% (if not a little more) in the majority of patients with baseline elevated heart rates. However, tachycardic patients can prove to be poorly responsive (or poorly tolerant) of β-blocker therapy, and these patients often require high doses. Medications that also might increase heart rate (particularly antihypertensive medications, ie, hydralazine, minoxidil, peripheral α-blockers) should be used sparingly in tachycardic patients unless accompanied by β-blocker therapy. In patients receiving nonspecific vasodilator therapy (ie, hydralazine, minoxidil), β-blocker therapy should, whenever possible, coincide with the timing of the vasodilator.

3. Does cardioselectivity and intrinsic sympathomimetic activity matter in the choice of a β-blocker?

β-Blockers may be classified as selective or nonselective, according to their relative abilities to block β_1 receptors (cardioselective) or β_1- and β_2-adrenergic receptors (noncardioselective). Cardioselective β-blockers include atenolol, betaxolol (Kerlone®), bisoprolol (Zebeta®), metoprolol (Lopressor®, Toprol-XL®), and nebivolol (Bystolic®). Receptor selectivity has been used as a marketing theme for several β-blockers, but the clinical relevance of this property remains uncertain. When used in low doses (eg, metoprolol 25 mg/day), β_1-adrenergic blocking agents preferentially block cardiac β_1 receptors with a lesser effect on the β_2 receptors in bronchial and vascular smooth muscle. In higher doses, (eg, metoprolol ≥50 mg/day), the β_1-selective agents lose their selectivity and also block β_2 receptors. Accordingly, β_1-selective agents are marginally safer than noncardioselective agents in patients with asthma and probably should be completely avoided in patients with severe, recurrent asthmatic attacks. In addition, low doses of β_1-selective agents offer a theoretic advantage in patients with peripheral artery disease (PAD) in that the β_2-receptors that mediate arteriolar dilatation may be unblocked; however, this effect has not been definitively shown.

Certain β-blockers, including acebutolol (Sectral®) and pindolol (Visken®), are actually partial agonists (termed intrinsic sympathomimetic activity [ISA]) that can bind to β_1- and/or β_2-adrenergic receptors. This combined effect (antagonist and partial agonist) has a neutral effect on heart rate when the sympathetic nervous system (SNS) is quiescent (ie, at rest), and there is a blunting of the expected tachycardic response with exercise. Acebutolol and pindolol appear to be as efficacious in reducing blood pressure or treating effort angina as β-blockers without ISA; however, these drugs do not provide the same level of cardioprotection in the post-MI patient—a circumstance in which cardioprotection is closely linked to the degree that the heart rate is reduced.

4. Does a β-blocker with α-blocking properties have any advantage over a regular β-blocker?

Despite pharmacologic heterogeneity, atenolol, carvedilol (Coreg®, Coreg CR™) (short- and long-acting formulations), labetalol (Trandate®), metoprolol (short- and long-acting formulations), propranolol, and timolol are all equally effective in the treatment of hypertension, despite the fact that β-blockers differ greatly with respect to their pharmacology (particularly in their receptor biology and important ancillary actions), hemodynamic effects, and tolerability.

Carvedilol, a vasodilating compound, is distinctive among β-blockers in that it is generally not associated with carbohydrate/lipid disturbances or weight gain. This agent has a neutral or beneficial effect upon insulin resistance, lipoprotein lipase activity, and levels of triglycerides (Tgs) and cholesterol, making it a useful option for the treatment of hypertension in patients with diabetes. This profile is also of some relevance in that these metabolic perturbations are factors that may underlie the failure of first- and second-generation β-blockers to effectively reduce cardiovascular morbidity and mortality. Until recently, carvedilol was only available as an immediate-release formulation requiring it to be dosed twice daily. A controlled-release (Coreg CR™) delivery system for carvedilol is now available, which allows once-daily dosing with maintenance of the favorable pharmacodynamic features of this compound.

5. To what degree are third-generation β-blockers, ie, nebivolol, different from first- and second-generation compounds?

Nebivolol, a highly lipophilic agent without ISA, is a β-adrenergic-blocking drug that combines a high degree of β_1 selectivity with endothelium-dependent vasodilating effects. Studies in normotensive and hypertensive patients have noted that nebivolol moderates nitric oxide (NO) release (and its bioavailability) within the vascular bed, thereby promoting vasodilation and reducing peripheral vascular resistance. A number of studies have consistently shown that nebivolol increases stroke volume, maintains cardiac output during exercise, and decreases central aortic pressure (unlike other β-blockers, ie, atenolol). This hemodynamic profile distinguishes nebivolol from other cardioselective β-blockers. Nebivolol generally also has neutral effects on carbohydrate metabolism and insulin sensitivity compared with other β-blockers. The frequency of sexual dysfunction and central nervous system (CNS) abnormalities (ie, fatigue, depression) with nebivolol are no different than what occurs with placebo. This low incidence of adverse side effects with nebivolol may relate to its being both highly selective for the β_1 receptor as well as its having a NO-mediated vasodilatory effect. Despite the favorable hemodynamic and tolerance profile of nebivolol, additional clinical trials are needed to determine the extent to which clinical events are reduced with this compound compared with conventional nonvasodilating β-blockers.

6. Should β-blockers be routinely used in the perioperative setting?

The American College of Cardiology/American Heart Association (ACC/AHA) 2006 Guideline Update on perioperative β-blocker therapy is the recognized position statement on the use of β-blockers in the perioperative setting. Class I recommendations (general agreement that the therapy is beneficial, useful, and effective) state that (1) β-blockers should be continued in patients undergoing surgery who are receiving β-blockers to treat angina, symptomatic arrhythmias, hypertension, or other ACC/AHA class I guideline indications and (2) β-blockers should also be given to patients at presumed high cardiac risk who are undergoing vascular surgery based on the finding of ischemia in preoperative testing. However, patients with decompensated heart failure, nonischemic cardiomyopathy, high-degree atrioventricular (AV) block, or severe valvular heart disease in the absence of coronary heart disease (CHD) should be cautiously (if at all) given β-blockers.

The optimal protocol for administration of perioperative β-blockers remains undecided. Few studies have compared different β-blockers, or distinguished their dose effect in the perioperative setting. Even fewer studies have included a titration scheme to the desired effect (eg, target heart rate) or investigated regimens that contain a preoperative trial of β-blocker therapy. Studies to determine the ideal target population, dose (and route), frequency of dosing, and dose limiting on-treatment blood-pressure values have not been undertaken.

The uncertainty concerning the answers to many of these questions is illustrated by the findings from the Perioperative Ischemic Evaluation (POISE) trial in which patients undergoing elective noncardiac surgery (age ≥45 years) with either vascular disease or multiple risk factors for cardiovascular events were randomized to metoprolol controlled release or placebo. Metoprolol was administered in a dose of 100 mg in the preoperative period, 100 mg in the 6-hour postoperative period, 200 mg 12 hours later, and 200 mg daily thereafter for 30 days. Doses were not adjusted unless systolic blood pressure fell <100 mm Hg, in which case the drug was stopped. With this β-blocker dosing scheme, the risk for nonfatal MI, revascularization, and atrial fibrillation was reduced; however, the risk for total mortality, stroke, significant hypotension, and bradycardia increased.

The findings from the POISE trial raise legitimate concerns about the routine perioperative use of β-blocker therapy in the patient undergoing noncardiac surgery. With such concerns, the available evidence (albeit less than definitive) suggests, whenever possible, that β-blockers should be started days to weeks prior to elective surgery, with the dose gradually increased until a resting heart rate between 50 and 60 beats/min is reached. β-Blocker therapy should continue during the intraoperative and postoperative period to maintain the heart rate <80 beats/min.

7. Are there any drug/drug interactions with β-blockers that are clinically important?

Patients with cardiovascular disease (CVD) often receive multiple concurrent therapies in addition to a β-blocker.

Such a scenario increases the opportunity for drug/drug interactions. Such interactions can be of a pharmacokinetic (resulting in a reduction or an increase in drug elimination) or a pharmacodynamic (due to the primary mechanism of the administered drugs) nature. Pharmacokinetic interactions can be either due to interactions at the point of drug-metabolizing enzymes (ie, cytochrome P450 [CYP450] enzymes) or at the level of drug transporter proteins, ie, P-glycoprotein.

6

An example of a β-blocker pharmacokinetic interaction is when a β-blocker is used with cimetidine (Tagamet®) (nonspecific CYP450 inhibitor), which is reported to increase labetalol, metoprolol, and propranolol (CYP450-metabolized β-blockers) levels by as much as twofold, but not change the level of the renally cleared β-blockers atenolol, nadolol, and pindolol. The concomitant administration of the antihistamine diphenhydramine (CYP2D6 inhibitor) with metoprolol (metabolized by CYP2D6) prolongs the negative chronotropic and inotropic effects of metoprolol in extensive (but not poor) metabolizers. A similar increase in metoprolol effect has been described with the co-administration of the selective serotonin reuptake inhibitor (SSRI) fluoxetine (Prozac®, Sarafem®) (CYP2D6 inhibitor). Carvedilol also has been shown to considerably raise the concentration of cyclosporin by inhibiting intestinal P-glycoprotein-mediated transport (decreasing absorption) of cyclosporin.

An example of a pharmacodynamic interaction in this drug class is the exaggeration in negative inotropic and chronotropic effects of diltiazem (Cardizem®, Cartia XT®, Diltzac®, Tiazac®) and verapamil (Calan®, Covera-HS®, Isoptin® SR, Verelan®) when given together with a β-blocker. Another example of the pharmacodynamic interaction is the attenuation of the antihypertensive effect of a β-blocker when co-administered with a nonsteroidal anti-inflammatory drug (NSAID). Finally, abrupt withdrawal of clonidine (Catapres®) while receiving a β-blocker may exaggerate the rebound hypertension due to unopposed α-stimulation. α-/β-Blockers (ie, labetalol) may prevent the occurrence of rebound hypertension.

8. What are the metabolic consequences of β-blocker therapy?

Several factors limit the use of β-blockers in patients with diabetes and hypertension because β-blockers can worsen dyslipidemia and/or decrease insulin sensitivity. Most β-blockers adversely affect carbohydrate and lipid metabolism, which may detract from their generally beneficial effect of blood-pressure reduction. Several studies have reported an increased incidence of new-onset diabetes and proatherogenic serum-lipid changes in patients with hypertension who were treated with β-blockers and/or thiazide diuretics. For example, in the Atherosclerosis Risk in Communities (ARIC) study, patients with hypertension who were treated with β-blockers had a 28% higher risk of developing new-onset diabetes.

Additional supporting evidence for an increase in the rate of new-onset diabetes with β-blockers was seen in two studies in which atenolol was the β-blocker used—the recent Anglo-Scandinavian Cardiac Outcomes Trial-Blood Pressure Lowering Arm (ASCOT-BPLA) trial, and the Losartan Intervention for Endpoint Reduction in Hypertension (LIFE) trial. In the latter trial, atenolol-treated patients experienced a 25% greater risk of new-onset diabetes compared with those who received the ARB losartan (Cozaar®).

The original observations concerning the occurrence of new-onset diabetes with β-blockers were obtained from metabolic studies conducted in hypertensive patients treated with the cardioselective β-blockers atenolol and metoprolol. Long-term use of these β-blockers significantly decreased insulin sensitivity and glucose uptake, increased serum Tg levels, and lowered high-density lipoprotein cholesterol (HDL-C) levels. The weight gain that occurs with β-blocker therapy is an additional consideration with regard to new-onset diabetes. Nondiabetic hypertensives also present with the same β-blocker-related metabolic disturbances as described above. There are more than a few ways to minimize the adverse lipid and glucose effects seen with a β-blocker including using low-dose therapy, converting to a β-blocker with ISA, or switching to a β-blocker with α-blocking properties. Utilizing such treatment options is critical for metabolic syndrome patients because glucose intolerance and lipid abnormalities often exist before β-blocker therapy is initiated.

9. Is weight gain an important adverse side effect of β-blocker therapy?

Increased body weight is a clinical problem in the majority of patients with hypertension and in nearly all patients with type 2 diabetes and hypertension. Drugs, ie, β-blockers, that either cause weight gain through body fat accumulation or make it difficult for patients to lose weight are of particular concern in the diabetic population. In that regard, a systematic analysis has been performed on eight randomized, controlled hypertension trials involving 7,048 patients (3,205 receiving β-blocker therapy [first and second generation]) followed over a period ranging from 6 months to 10 years. There was a greater average weight gain (>1.2 kg) in β-blocker-treated patients compared with control subjects, with the majority of the weight gain taking place within the first few months of starting β-blocker therapy.

The effect on body weight with β-blockers can, in large measure, be explained by changes in various aspects of energy metabolism (<5% to 10% [which corresponds to 100 to 200 kcal/day]) including, but not limited to, a decrease in the thermogenic response to meals. β-Blockers may also negatively affect total energy expenditure by producing feelings of tiredness and decreasing anxiety. Such neuropsychiatric effects reduce so-called purposeless movement or fidgeting, which expend calories. Systemic β-blockade may also promote weight gain by inhibiting β-agonist-induced lipolysis.

This feature would make it more difficult for individuals to lose weight when using β-blockers. Finally, β-blockers have negative effects on exercise capacity, which should also be accounted for when these compounds are given to physically active hypertensive patients. Combination α-/β-blockers, ie, carvedilol, appear to be accompanied by less weight gain than what occurs with pure β-blockers, ie, metoprolol.

10. Are there any systemic effects with intraophthalmically administered β-blockers?

The most commonly used agents in the therapy of glaucoma are topically applied β-adrenergic antagonists. The formation of aqueous humor in the ciliary body is partially mediated by tonic sympathetic stimulation; thus, it is the basis for the one-third reduction in aqueous humor formation in response to β-adrenergic antagonist ophthalmic therapy. Ophthalmically administered medications are not just locally active because these drugs can gain access to the patient's systemic circulation. A substantial fraction of an ophthalmically administered medication can pass down the nasolacrimal duct ultimately to be systemically absorbed.

The issues with topical β-blockade and cardiovascular medicine are multiple and include recognition of the frequency with which topical β-blockade is employed, an understanding of the fractional volume of an administered drop that can be systemically absorbed, and the likelihood of a patient being inherently sensitive to β-blockade.

Extreme caution should be exercised with the use of topical β-blockers in patients in whom β-blockade poses a significant health risk. Most topical β-adrenergic antagonists in common use, with the exception of betaxolol, are noncardioselective and, therefore, block both β_1- and β_2-adrenergic receptors.

A number of adverse pulmonary sequelae also can follow from β-adrenergic antagonist ophthalmic therapy. These untoward consequences can range from a simple worsening of asthmatic symptoms to bronchospasm to respiratory failure and death attributable to bronchospastic complications. The fact that potentially serious cardiovascular complications may arise from topical β-blockade is underappreciated. The cardiac effects of topical β-blockade can range from a reduction in heart rate to bradyarrhythmias. Topical β-blockers can also influence daytime blood pressure, especially in those patients who are susceptible to the antihypertensive effects of β-blockers. Of even more interest is the observation that topical β-blockade may inadvertently lower nocturnal blood pressure.

Suggested Readings

Bangalore S, Messerli FH, Kostis JB, et al: Cardiovascular protection using beta-blockers: a critical review of the evidence. *J Am Coll Cardiol* 2007;50:563-572.

Bradley HA, Wiysonge CS, Volmink JA, et al: How strong is the evidence for use of beta-blockers as first-line therapy for hypertension? Systematic review and meta-analysis. *J Hypertens* 2006;24:2131-2141.

Brodde OE, Kroemer HK: Drug-drug interactions of beta-adrenoceptor blockers. *Arzneimittelforschung* 2003;53:814-822.

Cutler JA, Davis BR: Thiazide-type diuretics and beta-adrenergic blockers as first-line drug treatments for hypertension. *Circulation* 2008;117:2691-2704.

Fleisher LA, Beckman JA, Brown KA, et al: ACC/AHA 2006 guideline update on perioperative cardiovascular evaluation for noncardiac surgery: focused update on perioperative beta-blocker therapy: a report of the American College of Cardiology/American Heart Association Task Force on Practice Guidelines (Writing Committee to Update the 2002 Guidelines on Perioperative Cardiovascular Evaluation for Noncardiac Surgery): developed in collaboration with the American Society of Echocardiography, American Society of Nuclear Cardiology, Heart Rhythm Society, Society of Cardiovascular Anesthesiologists, Society for Cardiovascular Angiography and Interventions, and Society for Vascular Medicine and Biology. *Circulation* 2006;113:2662-2674.

Frishman WH, Alwarshetty M: Beta-adrenergic blockers in systemic hypertension: pharmacokinetic considerations related to the current guidelines. *Clin Pharmacokinet* 2002;41:505-516.

Hart PD, Bakris GL: Should beta-blockers be used to control hypertension in people with chronic kidney disease? *Semin Nephrol* 2007;27:555-564.

Leslie WS, Hankey CR, Lean ME: Weight gain as an adverse effect of some commonly prescribed drugs: a systematic review. *QJM* 2007;100:395-404.

Mancia G, Grassi G, Zanchetti A: New-onset diabetes and antihypertensive drugs. *J Hypertens* 2006;24:3-10.

Messerli FH, Bangalore S, Julius S: Risk/benefit assessment of beta-blockers and diuretics precludes their use for first-line therapy in hypertension. *Circulation* 2008;117:2706-2715.

Pedersen ME, Cockcroft JR: The vasodilatory beta-blockers. *Curr Hypertens Rep* 2007;9:269-277.

Sica DA: Current concepts of pharmacotherapy in hypertension—ophthalmically administered beta blockers and their cardiopulmonary effects. *J Clin Hypertens (Greenwich)* 2001;3:175-178.

Chapter 7

Calcium Antagonists

Calcium antagonists, or calcium-channel blockers (CCBs), belong to a structurally and pharmacologically diverse group of medicines that are grouped into three major subclasses—phenylalkylamines, benzodiazepines, and dihydropyridines. The prototypes of these subclasses are verapamil (Calan®, Covera-HS®, Isoptin® SR, Verelan®), diltiazem (Cardizem®, Cartia®, Dilacor® XR, Diltia®, Diltzac®, Tiazac®), and nifedipine (Adalat® CC, Procardia®, Procardia XL®), respectively. The pharmacologic mechanism of action for all CCBs is to decrease cellular calcium entry through the L-type calcium channel. CCBs uniformly reduce vascular resistance through this effect, and they have a diverse biological profile due to the ubiquitous presence of L-type calcium channels in a variety of tissues. The CCB subtypes have differential selectivity of action, which may explain why they vary considerably in their effects on myocardial contractility, sinus and atrioventricular (AV) node conduction, and regional vascular beds. Consequently, it is of interest to evaluate this heterogeneity, keeping in mind the effect of CCBs on blood pressure, their impact on reducing the incidence of cardiovascular (CVD) and renal disease progression, and possible side effects. This subclass of drugs is popular in clinical practice due to the fact that CCBs are effective in reducing blood pressure regardless of age, gender, ethnicity, salt intake, and even with concomitant nonsteroidal anti-inflammatory drug (NSAID) use.

Frequently Asked Questions

1. Are there differences between nondihydropyridine CCBs (NCCBs) and dihydropyridine CCBs (DCCBs) with regard to their ability to lower blood pressure?

All CCBs, if dosed appropriately, provide similar degrees of blood-pressure reduction. This is true whether you are using dihydropyridines, ie, nifedipine (30 to 90 mg), amlodipine (Norvasc®) (2.5 to 10 mg), or nondihydropyridines, ie, verapamil (120 to 480 mg), diltiazem (180 to 540 mg). However, the limiting feature for dosing CCBs may be related to tolerability because all of these drugs have a somewhat different tolerability profile. Consequently, the ability to control blood pressure at the highest doses may be limited.

2. Are there differences in tolerability between NCCBs and DCCBs?

This is an important concern as these drugs do possess a dose-dependent ability to lower blood pressure, but that dose-dependent ability can lead to side effects. With regard to DCCBs, the most common limiting side effects are related to headache, flushing, and edema. These side effects are clearly dose dependent and may limit the use of a fully therapeutic dose in some patients. The NCCBs diltiazem and verapamil have a somewhat different tolerability profile. Although they can cause edema, it is often not to the extent seen with DCCBs. With verapamil, constipation is not uncommon as the dose is escalated, whereas with diltiazem, occasionally nausea and fatigue may occur. Consequently, individualization is critical.

3. Are there differences in CCBs with regard to their ability to reduce cardiovascular end points?

All of the major subtypes of CCBs have been studied in large clinical trials involving cardiovascular end points. Because these drugs are often associated with robust reductions in blood pressure, invariably there is a lesser likelihood of myocardial infarction (MI), angina, and stroke. However, CCBs, particularly when used as a monotherapy, may be associated with an increased risk of plasma-volume overload and congestive heart failure (CHF) compared with other commonly used therapies, ie, diuretics or drugs that block the renin-angiotensin-aldosterone system (RAAS). But the NCCBs verapamil and diltiazem, due to their negative chronotropic effects, may slow the heart rate in patients with coronary disease, which could be beneficial. DCCBs usually do not affect heart rate, and thus have not been studied as primary therapies in post-MI patients. All CCBs possess anti-anginal properties.

4. Do CCBs act the same with regard to changes in urinary albumin excretion (UAE)?

It is evident from clinical trials that the NCCBs, when used as monotherapy, are more capable of reducing proteinuria compared with DCCBs. A recent systematic review of all published trials on this topic effectively illustrates this point. However, these drugs are often paired with a drug that blocks the RAAS as part of a blood-pressure-lowering regimen in patients with renal disease. A more important question to ask is whether the differential antiproteinuric effects of these CCB subtypes are still evident despite concomitant RAAS blockade. Although there is some controversy in the literature, it is apparent that, regardless of the CCB used in conjunction with an angiotensin-receptor blocker (ARB) in proteinuric diabetics, there is no difference in the risk of progression to proteinuria or renal disease.

5. Can I use a CCB with a β-blocker?

It is safe to use a DCCB with a β-blocker because there will be a minimal effect on the cardiac reduction system. But there is concern that higher doses of NCCBs and β-blockers may impede AV node conduction, increasing the risk for heart block. Consequently, it is advisable not to use an NCCB and β-blocker combination to lower blood pressure.

6. What is the best way to attenuate edema that is associated with CCBs?

This is an important tolerability question as it is one of the most common side effects associated with higher doses of CCBs. However, this is unlikely to be related to salt and water retention because CCBs have intrinsic natriuretic properties. The majority of studies suggest that using a drug that blocks the RAAS, either an ACE inhibitor or an ARB, is the most effective way to attenuate edema associated with a CCB. The mechanism of reduction in edema with RAAS blocking drugs in patients taking CCBs is unknown. It is theorized that, because RAAS blocking drugs facilitate vasodilation, they may reduce capillary leakage caused by the powerful vasodilatory effects of CCBs on distal peripheral circulation arterioles, particularly in gravity-dependent areas (ie, feet, ankles). Interestingly, loop diuretics do not appear to lessen the edema. However, thiazide diuretics may have a modest effect on the edema perhaps due to their differential effects on plasma volume and vascular function—loop diuretics facilitate volume reduction as their predominant effect, whereas thiazide diuretics have a more modest effect on plasma volume and a more important vasodilatory effect on vascular beds.

7. Is there still a concern for MI when using a CCB?

Over the past few years, much of the concern about the relationship between CCB therapy and MI has dissipated. A large number of studies have demonstrated that the use of CCBs reduces the incidence of cardiovascular events as part of an effective blood-pressure-lowering regimen. We also now appreciate that there may be a differential risk for cardiovascular events between shorter-acting DCCBs when given sublingually, vs longer-acting DCCBs or NCCBs, as would be commonly prescribed for the control of hypertension. The shorter-acting drugs, because of a potential precipitous reduction in blood pressure, may be associated with an increased risk for cardiovascular events.

Suggested Readings

Agodoa LY, Appel L, Bakris GL, et al: Effect of ramipril vs amlodipine on renal outcomes in hypertensive nephrosclerosis: a randomized controlled trial. *JAMA* 2001;285:2719-2728.

Bakris GL, Weir MR, Secic M, et al: Differential effects of calcium antagonist subclasses on markers of nephropathy progression. *Kidney Int* 2004;65:1991-2002.

Effects of calcium antagonists on the risks of coronary heart disease, cancer and bleeding. Ad Hoc Subcommittee of the Liaison Committee of the World Health Organisation and the International Society of Hypertension. *J Hum Hypertens* 1997;11:331-342.

Lewis EJ, Hunsicker LG, Clarke WR, et al: Renoprotective effect of the angiotensin-receptor antagonist irbesartan in patients with nephropathy due to type 2 diabetes. *N Engl J Med* 2001;345: 851-860.

Materson BJ, Reda DJ, Cushman WC, et al: Single-drug therapy for hypertension in men. A comparison of six antihypertensive agents with placebo. The Department of Veterans Affairs Cooperative Study Group on Antihypertensive Agents. *N Engl J Med* 1993;328: 914-921.

Piepho RW, Culbertson VL, Rhodes RS: Drug interactions with the calcium-entry blockers. *Circulation* 1987;75(6 pt 2):V181-V194.

Saunders E, Weir MR, Kong BW, et al: A comparison of the efficacy and safety of a beta-blocker, a calcium channel blocker, and a converting enzyme inhibitor in hypertensive blacks. *Arch Intern Med* 1990;150:1707-1713.

Schrier RW, Estacio RO, Esler A, et al: Effects of aggressive blood pressure control in normotensive type 2 diabetic patients on albuminuria, retinopathy and strokes. *Kidney Int* 2002;61:1086-1097.

Chapter 8

ACE Inhibitors

Ten angiotensin-converting enzyme (ACE) inhibitors are currently marketed in the United States. Other than lisinopril (Prinivil®, Zestril®) and captopril (Capoten®), ACE inhibitors are given in their prodrug form, which enhances their absorption. ACE inhibitors are structurally heterogeneous, being distinguished by sulfhydryl (captopril), phosphinyl (fosinopril [Monopril®]), or carboxyl (all other ACE inhibitors) side groups. Although individual ACE inhibitors have differing absorption, protein and tissue binding, half-life, and mode of metabolic disposition, all drugs in this class similarly reduce blood pressure when comparable doses are administered. ACE inhibitors localize or bind to specific tissues, which may relate to their lipophilicity. Highly lipophilic ACE inhibitors, such as quinapril (Accupril®) and ramipril (Altace®), provide better 'tissue ACE' inhibition experimentally, an aspect of their action that is still of undetermined clinical importance.

Hypertension

ACE inhibition produces a variety of interlinked hemodynamic effects. In hypertension, there is a balanced reduction of cardiac preload (through the vasodilatory effects of ACE inhibitors) and afterload (through direct and indirect arterial dilator effects) with an ACE inhibitor. Because angiotensin II (Ang II) facilitates sympathetic nervous system (SNS) activation, ACE inhibition tends to limit stress-induced increases in catecholamines. ACE inhibition and its effect on blood pressure typically has no effect on heart rate.

Heart Failure

ACE inhibitor use improves the abnormal hemodynamics that define systolic forms of heart failure. Cardiac afterload is reduced because of both vasodilation and an improvement in large artery compliance. Stroke volume and ejection fraction (EF) often increase in the process of such hemodynamic changes as long as any therapy-related decrease in blood pressure is not excessive. Myocardial oxygen consumption is not increased, in part because ACE inhibitors also reduce cardiac preload and pulmonary wedge pressures by their venodilating effects.

Blood-Pressure Effects

The blood-pressure reduction with ACE inhibitor monotherapy is comparable to that of most other drug classes, with response rates from 40% to 70% in stages 1 and 2 hypertension. There are few pure predictors of response to an ACE inhibitor other than elevated plasma-renin activity (PRA) levels; however, in a general population setting, there is a limited relationship between PRA and the fall in blood pressure with an ACE inhibitor. On the basis of trials comparing trough-to-peak activity ratios with 24-hour ambulatory blood-pressure monitoring, several ACE inhibitors, including fosinopril, lisinopril, perindopril (Aceon®), ramipril, and trandolapril (Mavik®), can be administered once daily.

Frequently Asked Questions

1. Do certain patient subgroups have different response patterns to ACE inhibitors?

Certain patient subsets demonstrate lower response rates to ACE inhibitor monotherapy, including low-renin, salt-sensitive individuals, such as diabetic and black hypertensive patients. The low-renin state in elderly hypertensive patients is an exception in that it develops not as a result of volume expansion, although these patients are salt sensitive, but because of age-related decreases in plasma renin. The elderly generally respond adequately to ACE inhibitors, although interpretation of such a response is complicated by senescence-related renal failure causing a delay in the elimination of these typically renally cleared drugs. Black patients with hypertension are perceived as being less responsive to ACE inhibitors; this is correct when viewing the entire population but not on an individual basis. If adequate dose titration of an ACE inhibitor occurs, blood pressure can be effectively lowered in a certain number of patients who otherwise exhibit a suboptimal treatment response. Racial differences in blood-pressure response are normally eliminated when a diuretic is added to an ACE inhibitor.

2. What is the best way to determine the correct dose of an ACE inhibitor?

The question is often raised as to what to do if an ACE inhibitor fails to normalize blood pressure. One approach is to increase the dose; the dose-response curve for ACE inhibitor is steep at low doses and flat thereafter, but not as flat as had been previously believed. Dose titration helps to improve trough effects and prolong the duration of peak effect but has less impact on the peak blood-pressure effect itself. The duration of ACE inhibitor therapy also relates to the treatment response. The final blood-pressure response to an ACE inhibitor is generally not present until several weeks after therapy has been initiated. If a partial response to an ACE inhibitor has occurred, therapy can be continued at a particular dose in anticipation of an additional drop in blood pressure over the ensuing weeks because of vascular remodeling.

There is no evidence to support switching from an ACE inhibitor to an angiotensin-receptor blocker (ARB) if the

ACE inhibitor has failed. If ACE inhibitor therapy has decreased blood pressure (but not to goal), drugs that provide an additive (but not synergistic) effect for additional blood-pressure lowering include diuretics, calcium-channel blockers (CCBs), and peripheral α-blockers. In the case of each of these drug classes, the additional blood-pressure reduction seen occurs in a dose-dependent manner, particularly with diuretics. Diuretic doses as low as 6.25 mg of hydrochlorothiazide (Esidrix®, Microzide®) can evoke this additive response, suggesting that even subtle alterations in sodium balance are sufficient to boost the effect of an ACE inhibitor. The combination of an ACE inhibitor and an ARB is not significantly better for blood-pressure reduction than either given alone at maximum doses. Of note, among antihypertensive compounds used to treat hypertension, the incidence of new-onset diabetes appears to be the lowest with ACE inhibitors and ARBs.

3. Is there a class effect among ACE inhibitors?

ACE inhibitors all comparably reduce blood pressure if given in comparable doses; however, because there are few properties that truly separate one ACE inhibitor from another, cost has become progressively more relevant. Without a consensus definition on 'class effect,' this expression is often brought into play to legitimatize substituting one compound in a class for another, especially when a higher-priced agent has been purposely studied in a disease state such as heart failure or diabetic nephropathy. Relative to class effect for cardiovascular outcomes, it is uncertain what represents equivalent doses among ACE inhibitors. Therefore, although class effect is likely, there is no certainty that the correct dose of a substituted ACE inhibitor has been selected, particularly when favorable cardiovascular outcomes have occurred independent of measurable blood-pressure change, as in the case of ramipril in the Heart Outcomes Protection Evaluation (HOPE) study.

4. Is there an ideal dose of an ACE inhibitor for cardioprotection in high-risk coronary artery disease (CAD) patient?

In the HOPE study, low-dose ramipril (2.5 mg/day) was ineffective at preventing cardiovascular events, whereas a higher dose of ramipril (10 mg) provided considerable benefit. The European Trial on Reduction of Cardiac Events With Perindopril in Stable Coronary Artery Disease (EUROPA) showed that an 8 mg dose of perindopril is the appropriate cardioprotective dose for this compound. The results from EUROPA complement those observed in the HOPE study, and in the case of both of these studies, the dose of ramipril and perindopril used appeared not to have reduced blood pressure in a meaningful fashion. Higher doses of either compound would likely produce additional cardiovascular protection if for no other reason than blood pressure would be reduced.

Alternatively, the Prevention of Events with Angiotensin-Converting Enzyme Inhibition (PEACE) trial studied the effect of adding the ACE inhibitor trandolapril (4 mg) to a contemporary therapeutic regimen for patients with stable CAD and preserved left-ventricular (LV) function. In this study, the addition of trandolapril did not provide any additional benefit in terms of reducing the incidence of cardiovascular events. One possible explanation for the difference between these various studies is that the dose of trandolapril (4 mg) given was insufficient in the setting of what was an extremely-low-background event rate having evolved from the regular administration of other effective therapies (ie, aspirin, statins). Thus, in choosing the dose of an ACE inhibitor for the high-risk CAD patient, one should be mindful of the drug, the concomitant therapies, and whether the dose selected reduces blood pressure, which in and of itself will provide additional benefits.

5. Does an ARB provide the same cardiovascular benefits as an ACE inhibitor in ACE inhibitor-intolerant patients?

The Telmisartan Randomized Assessment Study in ACE Intolerant Subjects With Cardiovascular Disease (TRANSCEND) assessed whether the ARB telmisartan (Micardis®) (80 mg/day) provided end-organ protection in patients intolerant to ACE inhibitors with CVD or diabetes with end-organ damage. This study had a primary composite end point of cardiovascular death, myocardial infarction (MI), stroke, or hospitalization for heart failure. Telmisartan was well tolerated in patients unable to tolerate ACE inhibitors. Telmisartan did not affect the primary outcome in a statistically significant fashion; however, there was a clear reduction in the HOPE secondary outcome of cardiovascular death, MI, and stroke with telmisartan vs placebo. The inclusion of hospitalization for heart failure in the primary outcome of this study proved to be the undoing of this study. Future analyses of this trial will likely outline more clearly in which patient type the maximum benefit exists for use of the ARB telmisartan in ACE inhibitor-intolerant patients.

6. Does the combination of an ACE inhibitor and an ARB provide cardiovascular benefits beyond what would be seen with either drug class alone?

The ACE inhibitor ramipril (10 mg/day) and the ARB telmisartan (80 mg/day) were compared to combination therapy with both drugs in the Ongoing Telmisartan Alone and in Combination With Ramipril Global Endpoint Trial (ONTARGET). The primary composite end point of this study was death from cardiovascular causes, MI, stroke, or hospitalization for heart failure.

Although the mean blood pressure was slightly lower in the combination therapy group, there was no benefit seen beyond what was observed with ACE inhibitor or ARB therapy alone; thus, telmisartan was equivalent to ramipril in patients with vascular disease or high-risk diabetes and combination therapy was not better than either. Of note, combination therapy significantly increased the risk of hypotension, syncope, renal dysfunction, and hyperkalemia; thus, combination therapy with an ACE inhibitor and an ARB would appear to be ill advised because the benefit is exceeded by the risk.

7. How is ACE inhibitor-related hyperkalemia best managed?

ACE inhibitors and ARBs will increase the serum-potassium value in virtually all treated subjects but to a degree (0.1 to 0.2 mmol/L) that is not noticeable clinically. Clinically significant hyperkalemia with ACE inhibitors generally arises only in predisposed patients with a reduced glomerular filtration rate (GFR) or hypoaldosteronism (diabetics or heart failure patients with a reduced GFR). Use of potassium-sparing diuretics or potassium supplements increases the likelihood of hyperkalemia with an ACE inhibitor. Salt substitutes are enriched sources of potassium (60 mmol/tsp) and should always be considered as a 'hidden' source of potassium when an ACE inhibitor causes hyperkalemia. Nonsteroidal anti-inflammatory drugs (NSAIDs) and cyclooxygenase (COX) inhibitors also can exaggerate the rise in serum potassium seen with either an ACE inhibitor or an ARB by reducing aldosterone concentrations and thereby decreasing potassium excretion. It is uncommon even under the most extreme circumstances to see more than a 2 mmol/L increase in serum-potassium values with an ACE inhibitor or an ARB. When changes of this magnitude occur, it is generally in the setting of a sudden fall in GFR, prompted either by the ACE inhibitor or ARB (as is the case with renal artery stenosis or due to a volume-depleting intercurrent illness).

The frequency with which serum-potassium values should be monitored in an ACE inhibitor-treated patient should be based on pretherapy potassium values, the level of renal function, the presence of diabetes, whether concomitant medications are being given that might influence systemic potassium balance, and past occurrences of hyperkalemia. ACE inhibitor-/ARB-related hyperkalemia is class specific, not compound specific. There is scant evidence to suggest that one ACE inhibitor or ARB carries a lesser risk of hyperkalemia. If differences in the incidence of hyperkalemia truly exist among ACE inhibitors (or ARBs), as has been described for fosinopril, it is a phenomenon probably coupled to the absence of drug accumulation in chronic kidney disease (CKD) for certain ACE inhibitors. A final consideration is whether ARB therapy is associated with a lesser rate of hyperkalemia development than is the case for ACE inhibitors. In this regard, the absolute change in serum potassium with an ARB is somewhat less (0.1 to 0.3 mmol/L) than that observed with an ACE inhibitor.

8. How is a change in renal function approached in an ACE inhibitor-treated patient?

A form of functional renal insufficiency has been observed with ACE inhibitors in patients with either a solitary kidney and high-grade renal artery stenosis or bilateral renal artery stenosis. This phenomenon occurs more commonly when conditions of dehydration, heart failure, and microvascular renal disease are superimposed on large-vessel disease. The theme common to these conditions is one of reduced glomerular filtration pressures. When glomerular filtration pressures initially fall, intrarenal production of Ang II increases, which supports glomerular filtration by efferent arteriolar constriction. The abrupt removal of Ang II that occurs with ACE inhibitor therapy relaxes efferent arterioles and thereby reduces glomerular pressure to a level too low to maintain adequate filtration. A 25% increase in serum creatinine is a top-end change in renal function to be accepted in an ACE inhibitor- (or ARB-) treated patient before management or diagnostic steps are taken. Discontinuation of the ACE inhibitor (and restarting at a lower dose as therapy is warranted) or careful volume repletion (if the patient is volume contracted) typically corrects this problem. In the occasional patient, an increase in serum creatinine of this magnitude marks underlying renovascular disease and justifies a diagnostic work-up for this disease.

9. Is there a specific level of renal function at which an ACE inhibitor cannot be used?

There is not a specific level of renal function at which ACE inhibitor (or ARB) therapy is contraindicated. In fact, in most of the renal trials using either of these drug classes, the best results were seen with the higher starting serum-creatinine value. The typically small change in serum creatinine (10% to 15% increase from baseline) that occurs on starting an ACE inhibitor or an ARB is not a reason to stop or (in anticipation of such a change) not to start either an ACE inhibitor or an ARB. However, ACE inhibitor use in renal failure can be limited by unacceptable degrees of hyperkalemia; nevertheless, hyperkalemia can be managed in the ACE inhibitor-treated patient by careful control of dietary potassium intake, judicious use of diuretics, and the occasional administration of potassium-binding resins.

10. Is cough a class effect with ACE inhibitors?

A dry, irritating, nonproductive cough is a common complication with ACE inhibitors, with an incidence between 0% and 44%. Cough is a class phenomenon with ACE inhibitors and has ostensibly been attributed to an increase in bradykinin and/or other vasoactive peptides, such as Substance P, which may play a second messenger role in setting off the cough reflex. ACE inhibitor-related cough has been variably described as a risk factor for the likelihood of developing angioedema. Although numerous therapies have been tried, few have had any enduring success in eliminating ACE inhibitor-induced cough. The sensible clinical approach for suspected ACE inhibitor-related cough is to reassess the patient several weeks after drug discontinuation. Disappearance of the cough can then be taken as proof of an ACE inhibitor etiology. In most instances, there is no need to rechallenge a patient to irrefutably establish a cause and effect relationship between an ACE inhibitor and cough. In certain instances, ACE inhibitor-related cough is of some benefit in that its presence has been shown to decrease the risk of aspiration pneumonia, which has some bearing on the poststroke patient.

11. Can an ACE inhibitor-treated patient who develops angioedema receive an ARB?

Angioneurotic edema is an unpredictable and potentially life-threatening complication of ACE inhibitor therapy, which fortunately is uncommon, occurring in <1% of treated patients. It is about three times more common in blacks than in whites. Angioedema typically occurs shortly after beginning therapy with an ACE inhibitor, although it has also been seen years after beginning an ACE inhibitor, but rarely. Angioneurotic edema has a distinctive pattern of involvement with severe swelling of the mouth, tongue, and upper airway, and at its extreme, can be life threatening.

An ARB can be administered to a patient who has experienced previous ACE inhibitor-related angioedema if the patient is properly advised of the risk of recurrent angioedema. Despite the relatively benign nature of most angioedema episodes and the infrequency of cross-reactivity for angioedema with an ARB, these drugs still carry a discrete risk, albeit small, in patients having previously experienced angioedema with an ACE inhibitor. If ARB therapy is being considered in a patient with prior ACE inhibitor-related angioedema, there should be a reasonable justification for its use. Examples of patients for whom ARB use may be justified, when there had been a prior episode of ACE inhibitor-related angioedema, include patients with heart failure or proteinuric renal disease and those with a high cardiac risk.

12. Do ACE inhibitors have any effect on hemoglobin concentration?

A side effect associated with ACE inhibitors is anemia. ACE inhibitors (and ARBs) suppress the production of erythropoietin in a dose-dependent manner, which presents a particular problem when ACE inhibitors are administered in the presence of heart failure and/or CKD. ACE inhibitor-related anemia is, in part, related to N-acetyl-seryl-aspartyl-lysyl-proline buildup. This substance is mainly degraded by ACE and is a potent natural inhibitor of hematopoietic stem cell proliferation as well as an antifibrotic moiety. Because of the increase in N-acetyl-seryl-aspartyl-lysyl-proline concentrations with ACE inhibitor therapy, these compounds may be preferred for suppression of red cell production when it is a therapeutic goal. Such settings include posttransplant erythrocytosis, high-altitude polycythemia, cystic renal disease, and sleep apnea-related erythrocytosis. As much as a 4.5 g/dL fall in hemoglobin concentration has been observed with ACE inhibitor therapy.

Suggested Readings

Bakris GL, Weir MR: Angiotensin-converting enzyme inhibitor-associated elevations in serum creatinine: is this a cause for concern? *Arch Intern Med* 2000;160:685-693.

Casas JP, Chua W, Loukogeorgakis S, et al: Effect of inhibitors of the renin-angiotensin system and other antihypertensive drugs on renal outcomes: systematic review and meta-analysis. *Lancet* 2005;366:2026-2033.

Dzau VJ, Bernstein K, Celermajer D, et al: The relevance of tissue angiotensin-converting enzyme: manifestations in mechanistic and endpoint data. *Am J Cardiol* 2001;88:1L-20L.

Ersoy A, Kahvecioglu S, Ersoy C, et al: Anemia due to losartan in hypertensive renal transplant recipients without posttransplant erythrocytosis. *Transplant Proc* 2005;37:2148-2150.

Garg R, Yusuf S: Overview of randomized trials of angiotensin-converting enzyme inhibitors on mortality and morbidity in patients with heart failure. Collaborative Group on ACE Inhibitor Trials. *JAMA* 1995;273:1450-1456.

ONTARGET Investigators and Yusuf S, Teo KK, Pogue J, et al: Telmisartan, ramipril, or both in patients at high risk for vascular events. *N Engl J Med* 2008;358:1547-1559.

Schmieder RE, Hilgers KF, Schlaich MP, et al: Renin-angiotensin system and cardiovascular risk. *Lancet* 2007;369:1208-1219.

Schoolwerth AC, Sica DA, Ballermann BJ, et al: Renal considerations in angiotensin converting enzyme inhibitor therapy: a statement for healthcare professionals from the Council on the Kidney in Cardiovascular Disease and the Council for High Blood Pressure Research of the American Heart Association. *Circulation* 2001;104:1985-1991.

Sica DA: Angiotensin-converting enzyme inhibitors side effects—physiologic and non-physiologic considerations. *J Clin Hypertens (Greenwich)* 2004;6:410-416.

Sica DA, Black HR: Current concepts of pharmacotherapy in hypertension: ACE inhibitor-related angioedema: can angiotensin-receptor blockers be safely used? *J Clin Hypertens (Greenwich)* 2002;4:375-380.

The Telmisartan Randomised AssessmeNt Study in ACE iNtolerant subjects with cardiovascular Disease (TRANSCEND) Investigators: Effects of the angiotensin-receptor blocker telmisartan on cardiovascular events in high-risk patients intolerant to angiotensin-converting enzyme inhibitors: a randomised controlled trial. *Lancet* 2008 Aug 29;Epub ahead of publication.

Yusuf S, Sleight P, Pogue J, et al: Effects of an angiotensin-converting enzyme inhibitor, ramipril, on cardiovascular events in high-risk patients. The Heart Outcomes Prevention Evaluation Study Investigators. *N Engl J Med* 2000;342:145-153.

Chapter 9

Angiotensin-Receptor Blockade and Renal Protection

Prior to the introduction of angiotensin-receptor blockers (ARBs) for the treatment of hypertension, it was known for many years that angiotensin-converting enzyme (ACE) inhibitors were effective in not only lowering blood pressure and proteinuria, but also in providing renal protection for patients with nondiabetic renal disease and renal disease related to type 1 diabetes. Most of the ACE inhibitor renal protection studies were conducted with either captopril (Capoten®) or ramipril (Altace®), but the majority of ACE inhibitors also have comparable antihypertensive and antiproteinuric effects.

ARBs have similar blood-pressure-lowering effects as ACE inhibitors. They also have similar capabilities in reducing proteinuria. However, their mechanism of action is distinct compared with ACE inhibitors. The initial trials of these drugs to evaluate renal protection were conducted in patients with type 2 diabetes because no prior ACE inhibitor clinical trials had studied these patients. Based upon experimental data in animals, as well as the antihypertensive and antiproteinuric effects seen in humans, the assumption was that ARBs would have similar nephroprotective properties as seen with ACE inhibitors. Clinical trials have now been completed which demonstrate that ARBs are capable of delaying progression of microalbuminuria to clinical proteinuria, and progression of established diabetic renal disease to end-stage renal disease (ESRD).

The Irbesartan in Type 2 Diabetes and Microalbuminuria (IRMA-2) study evaluated increasing doses of irbesartan (Avapro®) (150 and 300 mg) or placebo plus other medications in 592 kidney patients with type 2 diabetes, hypertension, normal renal function, and microalbuminuria. The primary outcome of this study was time to manifestation of clinical proteinuria (>300 mg/day) over 2 years. The average blood pressure during the course of follow-up in each group was 144/83 mm Hg. Many patients required additional blood-pressure medications to reach goal (140/90 mm Hg). The highest dose of irbesartan (300 mg) resulted in a 70% reduction in the progression from microalbuminuria to clinical albuminuria compared with placebo. The 150 mg dose of irbesartan provided an intermediate benefit (39% reduction). The IRMA-2 study was the first study to show a blood-pressure-independent dose response to renin-angiotensin-aldosterone system (RAAS) blockade in patients with type 2 diabetes on the progression from microalbuminuria to clinical proteinuria.

Two large studies to evaluate possible nephroprotection of ARBs were contemporaneously performed in patients with type 2 diabetes, hypertension, an estimated glomerular filtration rate (eGFR) of about 50 mL/min/1.73 m^2, and clinical proteinuria. The plan for the Irbesartan Diabetic Nephropathy Trial (IDNT) (n=1,715) and the Reduction of Endpoints in NIDDM With Angiotensin II Antagonist Losartan (RENAAL) study (n=1,513) was to see whether angiotensin-receptor blockade as part of a similarly effective blood-pressure-lowering regimen could reduce the risk of the composite end point of doubling serum creatinine, ESRD, or death. In the IDNT, there were three treatment arms including a traditional approach of diuretic, β-blocker, vasodilator; an amlodipine (Norvasc®) (10 mg) arm plus additional drugs; and an irbesartan (300 mg) arm plus other drugs. Over the next 2.6 years, similar blood-pressure reduction occurred in all three groups to approximately 140/77 mm Hg. Despite similar degrees of blood-pressure reduction, however, those patients in the irbesartan group had a statistically significant reduction in risk for reaching the composite end point. Interestingly, the risk reduction for renal end points was entirely predictable based on the resultant change in proteinuria during follow-up. For every 50% reduction in proteinuria, there was a 50% reduction in renal events. Likewise, the RENAAL study compared whether the ARB losartan (Cozaar®) (100 mg) plus other drugs would be as effective or even more effective than a traditional non-ACE inhibitor blood-pressure-lowering regimen on a similar composite end point of renal failure and death as in the IDNT. After 3.4 years of follow-up, a similar, statistically significant reduction in risk for the composite end point, as well as the single end point of ESRD, was noted compared with traditional therapy. As in the IDNT, resultant proteinuria was important as a predictive measure of outcome for both cardiovascular and renal end points. These two studies established angiotensin-receptor blockade as the preferred therapeutic strategy as part of an effective blood-pressure-lowering regimen for type 2 diabetics to prevent the progression of both early- and late-stage renal disease.

Subsequently, the Diabetics Exposed to Telmisartan and Enalapril (DETAIL) study was performed to compare possible differences between the ARB telmisartan (Micardis®) and the ACE inhibitor enalapril (Vasotec®) on the rate of progression of renal disease in type 2 diabetics. Although only 136 patients were randomized in this study, the investigators did have 5 years of follow-up and conclusively demonstrated that there was no difference between an ARB or an ACE inhibitor regimen on the rate of progression of renal disease. Studies using other ARBs have demonstrated that ARBs have the clinically relevant capabilities of reducing blood pressure, microalbuminuria, and/or clinical proteinuria.

Frequently Asked Questions

1. Are all ARBS alike with regard to renal protection?

More likely than not, all ARBs provide a similar mechanism for their antihypertensive and antiproteinuric effects. However, there may be differences in pharmacology, duration of action, receptor binding, and other aspects of how the drugs function, which are not yet known. Whether these differences will prove to be important on slowing the rate of progression of renal disease is unknown. It is fair to say that evidence-based medicine supports the use of the dose of those ARBs that have been studied in the large renal protection trials as part of an effective blood-pressure-lowering regimen. The equivalent dose of other ARBs to provide renal protection is unknown, but it likely is the full dose approved for lowering blood pressure.

2. Are ACE inhibitors and ARBs the same with regard to renal protection?

The majority of data on ACE inhibitors has been gathered from patients with nondiabetic renal disease and in people with renal disease due to type 1 diabetes. The majority of data with ARBs has been gathered from patients with type 2 diabetes and nephropathy. The only study that has compared these drugs head to head is the DETAIL study, which demonstrated similar overall benefits. However, this study was small, and possible mechanistic differences between ACE inhibitors and ARBs may still prove to be important. As mentioned previously, evidence-based medicine supports the use of a therapy in the dose that was tested as part of a clinical trial with end points.

3. Is reduction of microalbuminuria or proteinuria the key factor in predicting renal protection?

This is a very intriguing question. To date, all of the available clinical trials that have evaluated resultant microalbuminuria or proteinuria during the course of a clinical trial have noted that renal disease and cardiovascular events track with the amount of microalbuminuria and proteinuria. It is important to note that not only is baseline microalbuminuria and proteinuria predictive of renal disease and cardiovascular events, but also time-varying microalbuminuria and proteinuria during the course of treatment. However, all of these studies were based upon secondary analysis of the clinical data. Thus, there is more interest now in performing prospective clinical trials to test the hypothesis that purposeful reduction of microalbuminuria or clinical proteinuria will result in fewer cardiovascular and renal end points. Thus, a change in albuminuria or proteinuria may serve as a biomeasure of the therapeutic success of a specific antihypertensive regimen.

4. Are there concerns about using ARBs in patients with higher levels of serum creatinine? Is there not a concern about changes in creatinine and potassium levels?

Patients entered the IDNT and RENAAL study with eGFR in the 50s and on average lost GFR at a rate of 3 to 5 mL/min/year. Thus, many patients finished the IDNT and RENAAL study with eGFR in the 30s or lower. However, only 1% to 2% of study patients had to have an ARB stopped due to changes in creatinine or potassium levels that the investigators felt were clinically significant.

Why does this discontinuation rate seem so low? In large part, changes in potassium were not uncommon. Yet, when the value was repeated, often hyperkalemia was no longer present. In addition, many of the patients were receiving concomitant loop diuretics, and the investigators made an effort to make sure that the patients were not taking salt substitutes or nonsteroidal anti-inflammatory drugs (NSAIDs). Changes in creatinine levels were also more common in the ARB groups. However, careful adjustment of diuretic support and avoidance of NSAIDs diminished the likelihood that patients would come off an ARB due to concerns about a rise in serum creatinine.

5. In these studies, was there an optimal level of blood pressure noted that was beneficial in slowing the progression of renal disease?

In the microalbuminuria studies, the progression of renal disease was slow. Consequently, there was little evidence to evaluate level of blood pressure on change in kidney function. However, those studies did demonstrate that reducing systolic blood pressure <140 mm Hg with different antihypertensive therapies reduced microalbuminuria. The benefits of lower blood pressure on the rate of progression of renal disease are more apparent in patients with overt renal disease as in the IDNT and RENAAL study. Secondary analysis of these studies demonstrated that levels of systolic blood pressure into the 120 to 130 mm Hg range were optimal for slowing the progression of renal disease. Moreover, even if one evaluated the type of pharmacotherapy used in these studies to lower blood pressure, it was apparent that RAAS blockade still provided important incremental risk reduction for renal and cardiovascular disease (CVD) events. Thus, both lower blood pressure, preferably into the 120 to 130 mm Hg systolic range, and blocking the RAAS with an ARB appeared to provide the greatest opportunity for renal protection.

Suggested Readings

Atkins RC, Briganti EM, Lewis JB, et al: Proteinuria reduction and progression to renal failure in patients with type 2 diabetes mellitus and overt nephropathy. *Am J Kidney Dis* 2005;45:281-287.

Bakris GL, Williams M, Dworkin L, et al: Preserving renal function in adults with hypertension and diabetes; a consensus approach. National Kidney Foundation Hypertension and Diabetes Executive Committees Working Group. *Am J Kidney Dis* 2000;36:646-661.

Barnett AH, Bain SC, Bouter P, et al, and the Diabetics Exposed to Telmisartan and Enalapril Study Group: Angiotensin-receptor blockade versus converting-enzyme inhibition in type 2 diabetes and nephropathy. *N Engl J Med* 2004;351:1952-1961.

Brenner BM, Cooper ME, de Zeeuw D, et al, and the RENAAL Study Investigators: Effects of losartan on renal and cardiovascular outcomes in patients with type 2 diabetes and nephropathy. *N Engl J Med* 2001;345(12);861-869.

de Zeeuw D, Remuzzi G, Parving HH, et al: Albuminuria, a therapeutic target for cardiovascular protection in type 2 diabetic patients with nephropathy. *Circulation* 2004;110:921-927.

de Zeeuw D, Remuzzi G, Parving HH, et al: Proteinuria, a target for renoprotection in patients with type 2 diabetic nephropathy: lessons from RENAAL. *Kidney Int* 2004;65:2309-2320.

Eijkelkamp WB, Zhang Z, Remuzzi G, et al: Albuminuria is a target for renoprotective therapy independent from blood pressure in patients with type 2 diabetic nephropathy: post hoc analysis from the Reduction of Endpoints in NIDDM with the Angiotensin II Antagonist Losartan (RENAAL) trial. *J Am Soc Nephrol* 2007;18:1540-1546.

Lewis EJ, Hunsicker LG, Clarke WR, et al, and the Collaborative Study Group: renoprotective effect of the angiotensin-receptor antagonist irbesartan in patients with nephropathy due to type 2 diabetes. *N Engl J Med* 2001;345:851-860.

Parving HH, Lehnert H, Brochner-Mortensen J, et al, and the Irbesartan in Patients with Type 2 Diabetes and Microalbuminuria Study Group: The effect of irbesartan on the development of diabetic nephropathy in patients with type 2 diabetes. *N Engl J Med* 2001; 345:870-878.

Pohl MA, Blumenthal S, Cordonnier DJ, et al: Independent and additive impact of blood pressure control and angiotensin II receptor blockade on renal outcomes in the irbesartan diabetic nephropathy trial: clinical implications and limitations. *J Am Soc Nephrol* 2005; 16:3027-3037.

Chapter 10

Renin Inhibitors

Renin inhibitors are a new therapeutic class of medications approved for the treatment of high blood pressure. The first available drug for clinical use, aliskiren (Tekturna®), was designed through a combination of molecular modeling techniques and crystal structure elucidation. It is an orally effective nonpeptide, low-molecular-weight chemical, which interferes with the first and rate-limiting step of the renin enzyme cascade. Aliskiren interacts with, and binds specifically to, the site of its only known substrate, angiotensinogen. This specificity of binding may provide more opportunity to limit the renin catalytic cascade because there is no reactive increase in plasma-renin activity (PRA), unlike angiotensin-converting enzyme (ACE) inhibitors or angiotensin-receptor blockers (ARBs). As a result, there may be more opportunity for rendering the renin system quiescent.

Aliskiren has low bioavailability (2.6%), yet it is effective in 150 and 300 mg strengths in reducing blood-pressure levels, and it has an effective half-life of >30 hours. Aliskiren is not actively metabolized by the liver, and it is excreted unchanged in the feces. Less than 10% of aliskiren is cleared by the kidneys. Consequently, dosage adjustment is not required in people with renal or hepatic impairment. Cytochrome P450 (CYP450) enzymes are not involved in the metabolism of this drug, which reduces the likelihood of most drug/drug interactions.

Clinical trials have demonstrated the dose-dependent efficacy of aliskiren in reducing both systolic and diastolic blood pressure. These studies show comparability in blood-pressure reduction to other commonly used antihypertensive drugs, ie, β-blockers, ACE inhibitors, ARBs. The tolerability of aliskiren is comparable with placebo, and it has a relative low incidence of adverse events with dosages tested in the 150 to 300 mg range.

Aliskiren has also been studied with other commonly used blood-pressure-lowering medications including amlodipine (Norvasc®), hydrochlorothiazide (Esidrix®, Microzide®), ramipril (Altace®), and valsartan (Diovan®). These studies illustrate the comparable additional systolic blood-pressure-lowering capability of aliskiren with all four therapeutic classes in the range of 5 to 7 mm Hg. Not only is aliskiren capable of neutralizing reactive increases in PRA and angiotensin peptides when used as monotherapy, but also when used in conjunction with other drugs, eg, hydrochlorothiazide, ACE inhibitors, ARBs.

Aliskiren has also been studied to evaluate changes in blood pressure after its discontinuation. Clinical investigation indicates that blood pressure remains reduced compared with baseline for 2 to 4 weeks after discontinuation. The explanation for this effect is unknown. However, it is unlikely to be related to the persistent effect of the drug within the circulatory system, given its half-life of 30 hours. Because aliskiren is highly tissue bound, particularly in the kidneys, there may be a persistent effect that influences sodium and water handling by the kidneys, which facilitates blood-pressure reduction.

Frequently Asked Questions

1. When should I use a renin inhibitor to lower blood pressure?

Clinical studies demonstrate that a renin inhibitor, ie, aliskiren, effectively reduces blood pressure to a similar degree as other commonly used drugs. It is also well tolerated and has placebo-like tolerability. Consequently, aliskiren is a useful therapy to be considered in the patient with essential hypertension. However, this drug has not yet been tested in specific clinical situations to evaluate its efficacy in reducing the risk of cardiovascular disease (CVD) or the progression of renal disease. Because ACE inhibitors and ARBs have been studied in numerous clinical trials with specific end points, these drugs remain the preferred choices for patients with evident heart or renal disease. However, since most patients require two or more medications to lower blood pressure, aliskiren may be a suitable choice to use with a thiazide diuretic, a calcium-channel blocker (CCB), an ACE inhibitor, or an ARB where there is a need of additional blood-pressure reduction.

2. Is a renin inhibitor the same thing as an ACE inhibitor or an ARB?

A renin inhibitor has a biochemically distinct mechanism of action compared with an ACE inhibitor or an ARB. ACE inhibitors interfere with the angiotensin-converting enzyme-1 (ACE1), which catalyzes the conversion of angiotensin I (Ang I) to angiotensin II (Ang II). As a result of this inhibition, there are also lower plasma levels of Ang I. However, there are also reactive increases in PRA and, subsequently, in Ang I. With long-term ACE inhibition, plasma Ang II levels rise back to and then above pretreatment baseline. ACE inhibitors also interfere with the breakdown of bradykinin. The accumulation of this vasodilator may also facilitate blood-pressure reduction, which may explain the increased frequency of cough associated with ACE inhibitor use.

ARBs are chemicals designed to interfere with the binding of Ang II to the AT_1 binding site, the preferred binding site of Ang II, known to influence many of the pathways that regulate blood pressure as well as vascular injury and repair responses. As a consequence of blocking the AT_1 receptor, there is a reactive increase in PRA, as well as in plasma

Ang I and Ang II levels. Whether the reactive rise of PRA or Ang I and Ang II levels as a consequence of ACE inhibition or angiotensin-receptor blockade is clinically significant is unknown. AT_1 receptor blockade may also shift the binding of Ang II to the AT_2 binding site. Theoretically, stimulation of the AT_2 binding site may facilitate vasodilatation and attenuate the proliferative effects of Ang II.

Aliskiren, a direct renin inhibitor, has no influence on the ACE or on the binding of Ang II to the AT_1 receptor site. Instead, it is a drug that binds to renin and interferes with the access of angiotensinogen to its binding site on renin, which inhibits the rate-limiting initial step of the RAAS cascade. As a consequence of renin inhibition, there is a similar blood-pressure reduction as one would see with an ACE inhibitor or an ARB, but renin inhibition has an entirely different biochemical picture. PRA, Ang I, and Ang II plasma levels decline with acute and chronic renin inhibition. Although the blood-pressure-lowering effects of aliskiren are comparable to other drugs, its biochemical effects on the RAAS cascade are completely different.

3. What are the most common side effects associated with renin inhibition?

Aliskiren, which is the first available renin inhibitor for clinical use, is well tolerated, based on clinical trial data involving about 10,000 patients. It has placebo-like tolerability that is comparable with an ARB. There do not appear to be any unique side effects associated with its use, except for the presence of diarrhea when doses >300 mg are used in human volunteers. Aliskiren does not appear to be associated with cough or angioedema to any greater extent compared with placebo, and it has modest effects on potassium homeostasis much like an ACE inhibitor or an ARB. A rise in serum potassium of 0.3 to 0.5 mEq/L should be expected. These increases can be greater if the patient receives drugs like potassium salts (ie, salt substitutes) or nonsteroidal anti-inflammatory drugs (NSAIDs). Modest increases in serum creatinine are also associated with renin inhibitors as well as with ACE inhibitors and ARBs. The increase in serum creatinine is 20% to 25%, and it is related to glomerular capillary pressure reduction. A greater reduction in the glomerular filtration rate (GFR) can occur if the patient is volume depleted, is taking NSAIDs, or has clinically significant renal artery stenosis.

4. Can you use a renin inhibitor with other blood-pressure-lowering drugs?

Clinical trials have shown that aliskiren works comparably with amlodipine, hydrochlorothiazide, ramipril, and valsartan in lowering blood pressure. The similarity of the blood-pressure-lowering effects in all four drug classes is interesting, and quite different than one would see using an ACE inhibitor and an ARB in combination where there is minimal incremental blood-pressure reduction. Perhaps this can be explained by the effect of the other renin-angiotensin-aldosterone system (RAAS) blocking drugs in increasing PRA as they lower blood pressure, whereas a renin inhibitor neutralizes this response. Using aliskiren with a β-blocker does not appear to improve blood-pressure reduction. This may be related to the fact that β-blockers have weak anti-renin activities, and, thus, may not compliment the more potent anti-renin activities of renin inhibitors.

5. Will dual RAAS blockade with a renin inhibitor and either an ACE inhibitor or an ARB provide more opportunity for the progression of cardiovascular (CVD) and renal disease?

This question may be one of the most interesting questions associated with the development of this new therapeutic class of blood-pressure-lowering medications. It is quite evident that ACE inhibition and angiotensin-receptor blockade have remarkably improved the ability (as part of a good blood-pressure-lowering regimen) to delay the progression of CVD and renal disease. However, these diseases still progress despite our best intervention efforts. Consequently, clinical trials have been undertaken (some completed and others ongoing) designed to evaluate whether dual RAAS blockade with a renin inhibitor and an ARB or an ACE inhibitor are preferable, compared with either therapy alone on intermediate measures of cardiovascular outcomes.

The Aliskiren Observation of Heart Failure Treatment (ALOFT) study assessed the effects of adding 150 mg of aliskiren (or placebo) to standard therapy (ACE inhibitor or ARB plus β-blocker) in patients with heart failure. Patients were clinically stable and received 3 months of treatment. Plasma N-terminal prohormone brain natriuretic peptide (NT proBNP) rose by 762 pg/mL in the placebo group and fell by 244 pg/mL in the aliskiren group. In addition, there was a fivefold greater fall in brain natriuretic peptide (BNP) in the aliskiren treatment group vs placebo. These favorable changes in BNP and NT proBNP have been associated with favorable cardiovascular outcomes in previous studies using ACE inhibitors and/or ARBs.

The Aliskiren in the Evaluation of Proteinuria in Diabetes (AVOID) study evaluated patients with type 2 diabetes and nephropathy who received 3 months of therapy with 100 mg daily of the ARB losartan (Cozaar®). Patients were then randomized to 6 months of therapy with aliskiren (150 mg daily for 3 months followed by an increase to 300 mg daily for another 3 months) or placebo in addition to losartan. In the aliskiren therapy arm, there was an additional 20% significant reduction in albuminuria compared with losartan and placebo. In addition, 25% of patients receiving aliskiren had a 50% reduction in albuminuria compared with 12.5% of those receiving placebo together with losartan. Although a reduction in urinary albumin excretion (UAE) correlates with slowing of progressive renal failure, the AVOID study did not evaluate this and ongoing renal outcomes studies with aliskiren are awaited on this point. Ongoing outcome studies of note with aliskiren include the Aliskiren in Visceral Obesity at Risk Patients Outcomes Research (AVIATOR) study, Aliskiren Trial in Type 2 Diabetic Nephropathy (ALTITUDE) study, and Safety and Efficacy of Aliskiren in Post Myocardial Infarction Patients (ASPIRE) study.

Suggested Readings

Azizi M, Menard J, Bissery A, et al: Pharmacologic demonstration of the synergistic effects of a combination of the renin inhibitor aliskiren and the AT1 receptor antagonist valsartan on the angiotensin II-renin feedback interruption. *J Am Soc Nephrol* 2004;15:3126-3133.

Azizi M, Webb R, Nussberger J, et al: Renin inhibition with aliskiren: where are we now, and where are we going? *J Hypertens* 2006;24: 243-256.

Brown MJ: Aliskiren. *Circulation* 2008;118:773-784.

Gradman AH, Kad R: Renin inhibition in hypertension. *J Am Coll Cardiol* 2008;51:519-528.

Gradman AH, Schmieder RE, Lins RL, et al: Aliskiren, a novel orally effective renin inhibitor, provides dose-dependent antihypertensive efficacy and placebo-like tolerability in hypertensive patients. *Circulation* 2005;111:1012-1018.

McMurray J, Pitt B, Latini R, et al: Effects of the oral direct renin inhibitor aliskiren in patients with symptomatic heart failure. *Circulation: Heart Failure* 2008;1:17-24.

Oparil S, Yarows SA, Patel S, et al: Dual inhibition of the renin system by aliskiren and valsartan. *Lancet* 2007;370:1126-1127.

Parving HH, Persson F, Lewis JB, et al, and AVOID Study Investigators: Aliskiren combined with losartan in type 2 diabetes and nephropathy. *N Engl J Med* 2008;358:2433-2446.

Pool JL, Schmieder RE, Azizi M, et al: Aliskiren, an orally effective renin inhibitor, provides antihypertensive efficacy alone and in combination with valsartan. *Am J Hypertens* 2007;20:11-20.

Sealey JE, Laragh JH: Aliskiren, the first renin inhibitor for treating hypertension: reactive renin secretion may limit its effectiveness. *Am J Hypertens* 2007;20:587-597.

Weir MR: Direct renin inhibitors: where will they fit in for antihypertensive treatment? *Curr Hypertens Rep* 2007;9:389-391.

Weir MR, Bush C, Anderson, et al: Antihypertensive efficacy, safety, and tolerability of the oral direct renin inhibitor aliskiren in patients with hypertension: a pooled analysis. *JASH* 2007;1;264-277.

Chapter 11

Aldosterone-Receptor Antagonism and Blood-Pressure Management

Two aldosterone-receptor antagonists (ARAs) are in common use in the United States—spironolactone (Aldactone®) and eplerenone (Inspra®). A third ARA, canrenone, is currently available in Europe. Although each of these compounds is comparably effective, structure/function relationships as well as metabolite/half-life considerations provide the basis for differentiating these drugs.

Spironolactone

Spironolactone was the first diuretic specifically engineered to oppose a renal transport process involved in sodium handling. Beyond the issue of efficacy, one must consider three aspects when judging the risk/benefit ratio of spironolactone—timing of effect, duration of action, and side-effect profile. Spironolactone's onset of action is characteristically slow, with a peak-response rate that can occur ≥48 hours after the initial dose. This lag time most likely occurs because spironolactone and, more importantly, its active metabolites (which have a long half-life) take several days to reach a steady state. The duration of the spironolactone effect may also differ substantially relative to natriuresis and antikaliuresis, with the latter often persisting for several days after its discontinuation. This outcome probably also relates to the extended half-life of spironolactone's metabolites. Structurally, spironolactone contains elements of the progesterone molecule and, as such, is not specific for the mineralocorticoid receptor. This explains its therapy-limiting progestogenic and anti-androgenic side effects (eg, gynecomastia, nipple tenderness, menstrual irregularities).

Eplerenone

The development of eplerenone was the result of a search to find an ARA with more specificity to block the mineralocorticoid receptor without its accompanying sexual side effects. Compared with spironolactone, eplerenone has up to a 500-fold lower affinity for androgen and progestin receptors, which translates into a several-fold decrease in adverse effects of a progestogenic and/or antiandrogenic adverse effects. Eplerenone has proven to be an effective antihypertensive compound as well as having an indication in the postmyocardial infarction (MI) patient with reduced systolic function.

Hypertension

The greatest positive hypertension treatment experience with ARAs is spironolactone, which has been used with or without a thiazide diuretic in the treatment of essential hypertension and more recently as add-on therapy for resistant hypertension. Of note, the mg-for-mg blood-pressure-lowering effect of eplerenone is less than that of spironolactone. The magnitude of the blood-pressure reduction with 50 mg of spironolactone administered twice daily is comparable to that seen with eplerenone administered 200 mg twice daily or 400 mg once daily, and is 1.3 to 2 times greater than that seen with eplerenone administered 50 mg twice daily or 100 mg once daily.

This add-on effect for blood-pressure reduction with spironolactone occurs within weeks, persists indefinitely, and occurs independently of ethnicity and urinary aldosterone excretion. When spironolactone (12.5 to 50 mg/day) was added to a regimen composed of a diuretic, an angiotensin-converting enzyme (ACE) inhibitor, or an angiotensin-receptor blocker (ARB), a mean decrease in blood pressure of 21 ± 20 /10 ± 14 mm Hg and 25 ± 20/12 ± 12 mm Hg was observed at 6 weeks and 6 months of therapy, respectively. The efficacy of aldosterone blockade in patients with resistant hypertension suggests that aldosterone excess (relative or absolute) may be a common cause of resistant hypertension.

Frequently Asked Questions

1. Which patient type is the best candidate for ARA therapy?

Clinical experience with spironolactone and eplerenone suggests these compounds are particularly effective antihypertensive agents in the low-renin hypertensive patient. There does not appear to be any gender-specific differences in response to these compounds. Spironolactone and eplerenone are often prescribed in combination with a kaliuretic diuretic to prevent hypokalemia and simultaneously obtain an additional hypotensive or natriuretic effect. Currently, spironolactone is used with some regularity in patients with resistant hypertension, with or without primary aldosteronism, who are receiving multidrug regimens that include a diuretic and any of several other drug classes, eg, an ACE inhibitor, an ARB, and/or a calcium-channel blocker (CCB).

2. What is the optimal dosing frequency for an ARA?

Spironolactone is usually administered once a day. There is no specific pharmacokinetic reason for twice-daily dosing of spironolactone, and one dose/day is as effective as multiple doses/day in hypertension. Considering the lengthy half-life of spironolactone (and its active metabolites) in patients with cirrhosis, the once-daily or alternate-day administration of spironolactone may be sufficient to generate adequate diuresis. If spironolactone therapy is deemed necessary for patients with renal failure, hyperkalemia can be a dose-limiting side effect. For patients with renal failure, spironolactone can be administered on an alternate-day basis to lessen exposure and the likelihood of hyperkalemia. In patients with hypertension, the initial starting dose of eplerenone is 50 mg/day. It is recommended that eplerenone be increased to 50 mg twice daily (and not 100 mg once daily) if blood pressure is inadequately controlled with the starting dose, as the antihypertensive effect of eplerenone is somewhat greater when it is administered twice daily.

3. Under what circumstances can ARAs be used as effective diuretics?

All ARAs are weak natriuretic agents when acutely administered to either normotensive or hypertensive patients. The natriuretic effect of these agents is greatest when aldosterone levels are high (primary or secondary hyperaldosteronism). This is particularly the case when spironolactone (eplerenone has not been similarly studied) is given to patients with cirrhosis and ascites or heart failure, circumstances in which secondary hyperaldosteronism is frequently present. Natriuretic effects with spironolactone are dose dependent and increase even as doses reach several hundred milligrams.

The diuretic effect of spironolactone takes several days to maximize, which likely relates to the time needed for its metabolites to reach a steady state. Spironolactone is of some utility in patients with cirrhosis and ascites because initial mild diuresis is sought, secondary hyperaldosteronism is clearly evident, and hypokalemia is particularly detrimental. ARAs, and spironolactone in particular, are useful adjunct agents when given together with diuretics working at more proximal nephron locations leading to their utility with thiazide and/or loop diuretics. This means of obtaining a diuretic response is conceptually termed sequential nephron blockade. A final consideration with spironolactone is that once therapy is discontinued its diuretic effect can persist for several days.

4. Is there a specific level of renal function at which an ARA should not be used?

Amiloride and triamterene (Dyrenium®) block sodium channels at the luminal membrane. For these drugs to work, they must be filtered and/or secreted to reach their locus of action. Accordingly, as renal failure advances, these compounds have progressively limited access to their site of action. Alternatively, spironolactone works on the basolateral membrane of tubular cells and does not rely on glomerular filtration or secretion to gain exposure to its site of action; thus, unlike amiloride, spironolactone can remain active even at fairly advanced stages of renal failure.

Spironolactone can be carefully used in renal failure with appropriate laboratory monitoring of serum potassium. The glomerular filtration rate (GFR) is a relative determinant of whether spironolactone can be used and should always be considered in the context of the prevailing serum-potassium value. For example, a patient with a GFR of 50 mL/min and a serum-potassium value of 5 mEq/L would be likely to develop therapy-limiting hyperkalemia with spironolactone; however, a different patient with a GFR of 30 mL/min and a serum-potassium value of 3.4 mEq/L could be cautiously treated with spironolactone. The Package Insert for spironolactone does not offer a specific level of renal failure at which this compound is contraindicated; thus, dosing in renal failure is discretionary to a certain degree. When spironolactone is used in the presence of renal failure, serum potassium should be monitored more frequently than in the nonrenal failure setting. Spironolactone-treated patients should be made aware of those circumstances likely to increase their serum potassium ie, volume contraction, nonsteroidal anti-inflammatory drug (NSAID) use, and/or an excessive intake of potassium.

5. Do ARAs have an effect on urinary protein excretion?

Both spironolactone and eplerenone have an antiproteinuric effect as monotherapy or when combined with an ACE inhibitor or ARB. Although the mechanistic basis for this antiproteinuric effect is uncertain, it appears to correlate with pretherapy aldosterone levels and/or the degree to which the GFR decreases with therapy. Of note, the antiproteinuric effect of these compounds is independent of any observed blood-pressure reduction and may be more prominent in patients with diabetic nephropathy. To date, spironolactone or eplerenone have not been specifically studied in chronic kidney disease (CKD) trials to determine if renal protection occurs beyond what is achieved with blood-pressure reduction alone.

6. Do ARAs have any effect on magnesium homeostasis?

Unlike other diuretics, ie, thiazide and loop diuretics, ARAs do not cause magnesium wasting, and they actually increase total body magnesium stores. The degree to which these compounds cause magnesium retention is a small fraction of the potassium retention they produce. The magnesium-sparing feature of these compounds is most evident when magnesium-wasting diuretics are used for volume control in either cirrhosis or heart failure. Whereas this magnesium-sparing property is of undefined significance in the patient with hypertension, it is a particularly useful feature in the patient with heart failure; therein the disease-state-related increase in aldosterone activity often leads to hypomagnesemia and an increased likelihood of arrhythmias. Even at low doses (about 25 mg/day), spironolactone can noticeably increase both plasma and erythrocyte magnesium, and thus reduce the risk of ventricular and atrial premature beats and atrial fibrillation/flutter.

7. *Does eplerenone have any active metabolites and is its metabolic profile clinically pertinent?*

Unlike spironolactone, no active metabolites have been identified for eplerenone. Eplerenone pharmacokinetics are not altered in a meaningful fashion in CKD, the elderly, or patients with hepatic dysfunction. The primary route of elimination for eplerenone is via cytochrome P450 (CYP450) 3A4-mediated metabolism; eplerenone does not, however, interfere with the metabolism of CYP3A4 substrates. Whereas spironolactone has a limited number of drug/drug interactions, eplerenone interacts with a number of medications. The metabolism of eplerenone can be slowed when coadministered with CYP3A4 inhibitors; thus, eplerenone should be administered with extreme caution (if at all) when potent inhibitors of the CYP3A4 system, such as ketoconazole (Nizoral®) and itraconazole (Sporanox®), are in use. In that regard, the area under the curve (AUC) for eplerenone increases fivefold when coadministered with ketoconazole. Less potent inhibitors of the CYP3A4 system, ie, erythromycin, verapamil (Calan®, Covera-HS®, Isoptin® SR, Verelan®) will double the AUC for eplerenone when chronically coadministered. The starting dose of eplerenone should be empirically reduced from 50 to 25 mg/day when such inhibitors are coadministered.

8. *Does spironolactone interfere with the analytical determination of other medications?*

Spironolactone is known to interfere with the analytical determination of digoxin (Lanoxin®) such that falsely low results can be observed. The mechanism underlying this interaction is suggested to be the structural similarity between digoxin, spironolactone, and canrenone (a spironolactone metabolite not available in the United States), as well as lesser spironolactone metabolites. Recently developed assays may be less prone to spironolactone interfering with digoxin measurement. This analytic interference may allow true toxic digoxin concentrations to go unrecognized and increase the chance of digoxin intoxication should its dosage be increased on the basis of falsely low values. Accordingly, physicians should familiarize themselves with the false-negative potential of the analytic method employed in their clinical setting. Absent such methodological familiarity, the extent of this interference can be minimized by sampling digoxin levels at a time farthest removed from spironolactone's administration.

9. What are the most common nonelectrolyte side effects that occur with spironolactone?

The most common side effect with spironolactone is that of breast complaints, with approximately 10% of males noting breast tenderness at a maximum dose of 50 mg/day. In general practice, this percentage is likely to be higher. Breast symptoms can include a symmetrical or asymmetrical increase in size (occasionally unilateral), the development of nipple and/or breast tenderness, and/or the appearance of discrete breast masses. Prior studies have found that the breast changes with spironolactone are dose dependent with a >50% incidence with spironolactone doses ≥150 mg. Gynecomastia is generally corrected upon discontinuation of the drug; however, the time required for reversibility can be prolonged particularly if gynecomastia is at an advanced stage. The nipple symptoms with spironolactone disappear before there is any reduction in breast size. Gynecomastia occurs much less frequently with eplerenone and it can be substituted for spironolactone in the patient with gynecomastia with the expectation that breast symptoms/structural change will remit over time.

10. How can hyperkalemia with ARAs be avoided or managed?

Spironolactone and eplerenone at doses of 25 and 50 mg, respectively, appear safe relative to the development of hyperkalemia as long as the background level of renal failure is not too severe. Typically, it takes 2 to 4 weeks to arrive at a stable state of potassium balance after beginning an ARA, which should be considered when serum-potassium values are obtained during therapy. Serum-potassium sampling should occur more regularly if an ARA is given in combination with either an ACE inhibitor or ARB. The circumstances that most commonly disrupt potassium homeostasis after a steady state has been reached for ARA effect are marked by rapid volume loss (and a reduction in GFR), ie, diarrhea or upper gastrointestinal (GI) illness. Under such circumstances, patients should discontinue ARA therapy until the intercurrent illness has resolved and the potassium status re-evaluated.

Several treatment options are available for hyperkalemia at these ARA doses. A number of these options should also be considered as pre-emptive therapies. Dietary changes that restrict potassium intake should be instituted and potassium supplements discontinued; patients should be questioned relative to the use of salt substitutes (about 60 mmol of potassium chloride/tsp). Combining an ARA with a potassium-losing diuretic may lower the baseline serum-potassium value; however, potassium-losing diuretics should only be used if diuretic-related volume losses do not reduce the GFR because this can significantly reduce urinary potassium excretion.

The dose of each compound can also be empirically reduced in the hyperkalemic ARA-treated patient, or the same dose can be given on an alternate-day basis.

It is unclear in the patient prone to hyperkalemia development whether simple dosage reduction is sufficient to correct this tendency. If spironolactone therapy is the basis for hyperkalemia development, then an empiric switch to eplerenone can be considered based on eplerenone's shorter half-life, however, head-to-head studies comparing equivalent doses of eplerenone and spironolactone for hyperkalemia risk have yet to be undertaken.

Suggested Readings

Calhoun DA: Low-dose aldosterone blockade as a new treatment paradigm for controlling resistant hypertension. *J Clin Hypertens (Greenwich)* 2007;9(1 suppl 1):19-24. Review.

Garthwaite SM, McMahon EG: The evolution of aldosterone antagonists. *Mol Cell Endocrinol* 2004;217:27-31.

Liew D, Krum H: Aldosterone receptor antagonists for hypertension: what do they offer? *Drugs* 2003;63:1963-1972.

Nishizaka MK, Zaman MA, Calhoun DA: Efficacy of low-dose spironolactone in subjects with resistant hypertension. *Am J Hypertens* 2003;16(11 pt 1):925-930.

Rose LI, Underwood RH, Newmark SR, et al: Pathophysiology of spironolactone-induced gynecomastia. *Ann Int Med* 1977;87:398-403.

Santos J, Planas R, Pardo A, et al: Spironolactone alone or in combination with furosemide in the treatment of moderate ascites in nonazotemic cirrhosis. A randomized comparative study of efficacy and safety. *J Hepatol* 2003;39:187-192.

Schjoedt KJ, Rossing K, Juhl TR, et al: Beneficial impact of spironolactone in diabetic nephropathy. *Kidney Int* 2005;68:2829-2836.

Sica DA: Pharmacokinetics and pharmacodynamics of mineralocorticoid blocking agents and their effects on potassium homeostasis. *Heart Fail Rev* 2005;10:23-29.

Sica DA, Hess M: Pharmacotherapy in congestive heart failure: aldosterone receptor antagonism: interface with hyperkalemia in heart failure. *Congest Heart Fail* 2004; 10:259-264.

Weinberger MH, White WB, Ruilope LM, et al: Effects of eplerenone versus losartan in patients with low-renin hypertension. *Am Heart J* 2005;150:426-433.

Chapter 12

Fixed-Dose Combination Therapy

Drug monotherapy is the preferred way to begin treatment of hypertension, although in many instances one drug alone is unable to bring blood pressure to goal even when maximally titrated. It is increasingly appreciated that the elusive goal of attaining a normal blood pressure is achieved only when multidrug therapy is employed. This is especially true when considered in the context of current lower blood-pressure goals.

The options for multidrug therapy are straightforward—either fixed-dose combination therapy or drugs added sequentially until an effective multidrug regimen is established. Although proponents exist for monotherapy and for multidrug therapy, there has been a shift toward more frequent use of fixed-dose, single-tablet combination therapy over the past decade.

A considerable legacy exists for fixed-dose combination therapies. Such therapy dates to the 1950s when reserpine and other rauwolfia derivatives were combined with other medications. For example, the combination of rauwolfia and the parasympathomimetic agent veratrum was marketed as Verapene®. The fixed-dose combination of reserpine and butalbital, marketed under the trade name, targeted the so-called anxiety/hypertension syndrome, in an era when anxiety and hypertension were considered as manifestations of sympathetic overactivity. A combination of reserpine/ephedrine employed ephedrine to counteract the psychoactive side effects of reserpine, supposedly without compromising the antihypertensive effect of reserpine.

The rationale for fixed-dose combination therapy has remained constant since the 1950s. Fixed-dose combination therapy successfully reduces blood pressure because two drugs, each typically working at a separate site, block different mechanistic pathways. In addition, the second drug of a two-drug combination may check counterregulatory system activity induced by the other. For example, a diuretic/β-blocker combination may find the diuretic correcting salt and water retention, which occasionally accompanies β-blocker therapy, or the combination of an angiotensin-converting enzyme (ACE) inhibitor/diuretic is complementary because the ACE inhibitor blocking renin-angiotensin-aldosterone system (RAAS) activity was prompted by the diuretic.

The side-effect pattern also differs with fixed-dose combination therapy because lower doses of the drug are often administered. In addition, the peripheral edema that accompanies calcium-channel blocker (CCB) therapy occurs less frequently when an ACE inhibitor or angiotensin-receptor blocker (ARB) is coadministered. ACE inhibitors and ARBs improve, if not completely eliminate, the peripheral edema experienced with CCBs because of their proven ability to venodilate. In addition, diuretic-induced volume contraction may cause secondary hyperaldosteronism as well as electrolyte abnormalities, ie, hypokalemia and/or hypomagnesemia. The coadministration of either an ACE inhibitor or ARB with a diuretic can often correct electrolyte disturbances.

In 2007, two single-pill combination drugs that combine amlodipine with either valsartan (Diovan®) or olmesartan medoxomil (Benicar®) were approved by the FDA for the treatment of hypertensive patients. The amlodipine and olmesartan medoxomil combination (Azor®) and amlodipine/valsartan (Exforge®) are approved for the treatment of hypertension in adults. In addition,

Exforge® is approved for the initial therapy of hypertension. Both combinations have been shown in clinical trials to significantly lower BP compared with the individual agents alone.

Frequently Asked Questions

1. What types of fixed-dose combinations are currently available?

Hypertension—Fixed-dose combinations are primarily available as products that contain a thiazide diuretic and any of several nondiuretic compounds, including ACE inhibitors, ARBs, centrally acting agents, and β-blockers. Thiazide diuretics have also been combined with a number of potassium-sparing diuretics, including amiloride, spironolactone (Aldactone®), and triamterene (Dyrenium®), but not eplerenone (Inspra®). There are currently no CCB/thiazide diuretic fixed-dose combinations on the US market. Almost all single-tablet combinations that contain a diuretic use hydrochlorothiazide (Esidrix®, Microzide®) and only a handful of products contain chlorthalidone (Thalitone®), eg, atenolol/chlorthalidone (Tenoretic®) and clonidine/chlorthalidone (Clorpres®). There are also no combination products that contain a loop diuretic on the US market. Diuretic-based, fixed-dose combinations typically contain from 6.25 to 25 mg of hydrochlorothiazide. In the United States, there are no fixed-dose products containing a β-blocker and a CCB. Globally, such combinations exist, eg, the β-blocker metoprolol (Lopressor®, Toprol-XL®), and the CCB felodipine (Plendil®). Several fixed-dose combinations containing either an ACE inhibitor or ARB together with a CCB are currently available in the United States. These combinations have proven to be fairly potent in their blood-pressure-lowering ability primarily because of the CCB component in the combination.

Hypertension and dyslipidemia—Hypertension and dyslipidemia are conditions that frequently coexist. In a recent study utilizing data from the Third National Health and Nutrition Examination Survey (NHANES III), it was estimated that almost 15% of the US adult population (representing about 30 million US adults) have both hypertension and dyslipidemia. In this analysis, >60% of patients with hypertension were also found to be dyslipidemic; conversely, about 50% of patients with dyslipidemia were also classified as hypertensive.

Hypertension and hypercholesterolemia are the two leading risk factors for heart disease, which is the leading cause of death worldwide. Presented together, these two disturbances result in an increase in coronary heart disease (CHD)-related events that exceed simple additive for expected event rates with each disease. The rather disappointing success rate (10%) for the simultaneous control of hypertension and dyslipidemia, in approximately 30 million Americans who have both of these disorders, offers an opportunity for alternative treatment strategies such as a newly available fixed combination of an antihypertensive and a lipid-lowering agent (amlodipine/atorvastatin [Caduet®]). 12

Of particular note, the amlodipine/atorvastatin combination drug should not be expected to substantially improve blood-pressure control beyond that accomplished with amlodipine alone and likewise for any additional cholesterol-lowering effect with amlodipine when administered with atorvastatin. Time will tell as to how physicians and/or patients embrace this therapeutic approach. Future combination drugs will expand treatment options and will likely employ other antihypertensive drug classes, ie, ACE inhibitors, ARBs, together with various other lipid-lowering agents. The arrival of these new combination products could pave the way for more expansive combinations that are not dissimilar to the recently proposed poly-pill.

2. Can dose titration with a fixed-dose combination therapy occur by simply giving two pills rather than one or must the components be individually titrated?

The answer to this question is probably yes. Many fixed-dose combination products use low doses of the individual components. A doubling of the medication dose, ie, two pills rather than one, would in most instances still provide a quantity of drug without the threshold for dose-dependent side effects being crossed. Whether such upward titration of medication best occurs by split dosing in the morning and evening, or is carried out by doubling the daytime dose is discretionary. Fixed-dose combination products have rarely been studied in a twice-daily dosing regimen.

3. Is blood pressure further reduced when the dose of a diuretic is increased in a fixed-dose combination product?

In the case of diuretic-containing, fixed-dose combination products, it has been believed for some time that lower diuretic doses effectively reduce blood pressure with dose-dependent side effects kept to a minimum. In this regard, fixed-dose combination therapies containing as little as 6.25 mg hydrochlorothiazide have been viewed as the standard for diuretic-containing combinations. However, a number of patients exhibit a progressive response to increasing doses of hydrochlorothiazide (≤50 mg). This is not unexpected because there is varying sensitivity to diuretic therapy in the hypertensive population; moreover, thiazide diuretics have a dose-dependent permissive effect on the action of several drug classes (ie, β-blockers, ACE inhibitors, ARBs). As a result, higher doses of a diuretic can be expected to improve the response to a number of nondiuretic antihypertensive medications, which is of particular importance in those patient subsets, ie, diabetes, chronic kidney disease (CKD), and high-risk coronary artery disease (CAD), with the lowest goal blood pressure.

The prescribing physician can provide additional amounts of diuretic in several ways. First, a separate prescription can be provided, however, this defeats the purpose of fixed-dose combination therapy. Second, the diuretic-containing combination product can be given more than once daily, unless multiple strengths of the fixed-dose combination product in question are available, which is the case for most products.

4. How does an ACE inhibitor and diuretic combination compare to that of an ACE inhibitor and a CCB relative to blood-pressure control and outcomes?

This question was addressed by the Avoiding Cardiovascular Events Through Combination Therapy in Patients Living With Systolic Hypertension (ACCOMPLISH) study. The ACCOMPLISH study compared the effects of two forms of antihypertensive combination therapies (benazepril/hydrochlorothiazide [Lotensin HCT®] and amlodipine/benazepril [Lotrel®]) on major fatal and nonfatal cardiovascular events in 11,400 subjects (systolic blood pressure ≥160 mm Hg or currently on antihypertensive therapy and with evidence of cardiovascular disease [CVD], renal disease, or target-organ damage). Patients enrolled in the trial were typically obese, with 60% having diabetes. The large majority of patients had been previously treated for hypertension (>70% had been treated with ≥2 hypertensive agents). At 36 months, blood-pressure levels were significantly improved with more than 75% of patients in both therapy arms achieving blood-pressure levels <140/90 mm Hg; however, the combination treatment with amlodipine/benazepril reduced cardiovascular morbidity and mortality (defined as cardiovascular death, fatal/nonfatal MI, fatal/nonfatal stroke, hospitalization for unstable angina [UA], and coronary revascularization) by 20%, compared with those treated with benazepril plus a diuretic. The results of the ACCOMPLISH study support the notion that a renin-angiotensin-aldosterone system (RAAS) blocker and a CCB should be considered more frequently as first-step therapies in the patient with hypertension.

5. Is there a circadian rhythm for the blood-pressure-lowering response associated with fixed-dose combination therapy?

A number of medication classes show evidence of a circadian rhythm for both their pharmacokinetics and pharmacodynamics. This is not surprising, especially if one recognizes the circadian pattern of many neurohumoral systems as well as the clockwise relationship of both blood pressure and renal function. This would predict a variable response to therapy according to the time of day that a drug or combination of drugs is administered. For example, administration of the ARB valsartan at bedtime vs upon awakening results in an improved day/night blood-pressure ratio, a significant increase in the percentage of controlled patients after treatment, and a significant reduction in urinary albumin excretion (UAE). Such a difference based on the time of day of administration likely relates, in part, to the fact that the RAAS is more active at night than in the morning or daytime.

The concept of a timewise response to pharmacotherapy becomes even more complex with the administration of single-tablet, fixed-dose combination therapy and, to date, a paucity of data exists that might offer insight into response patterns. If fixed-dose combination therapy is considered at points of time other than in the morning, careful observation should be used to identify the pattern of response. This is particularly the case with twice-daily dosing of a product containing either an ACE inhibitor or ARB because blood pressure may drop more with nighttime dosing of either of these drug classes.

6. Is compliance better with fixed-dose combination therapy?

A number of factors can be implicated in the failure of current therapeutic regimens to reduce blood pressure in a significant proportion of the US population, with medication compliance of the utmost importance. Despite decades of attention to medication noncompliance in treated hypertensive patients, this issue remains a significant factor in the inadequate control of blood pressure. Current approaches to enhancing compliance bring into play patient demographics, medication characteristics, clinical factors, health beliefs, and the quality of patient/provider communication. Compliant patients are commonly defined as those who take their medication on average at least 80% of the time. There are many patterns of noncompliance, which include taking less than the recommended dose, stopping medication completely, intermittently missing doses, and/or stopping their medication for several consecutive days in succession.

Fixed-dose combinations are designed to simplify the medication regimen, and, in so doing, potentially improve patient compliance. The comparison data on fixed-dose combinations with free-drug regimens to improve medication compliance is only now emerging. In that regard, a recent meta-analysis of fixed-dose combination with free-drug regimens found that the risk of medication noncompliance was decreased by 24% with a fixed-dose combination regimen. Market forces also now frequently dictate that the price of a fixed-dose combination product stays well below that of the individual components if purchased separately, which may be an additional determinant of compliance.

7. Can fixed-dose combination antihypertensive therapy be used as initial therapy in the treatment of hypertension?

There are a number of approaches to using antihypertensive medications in fixed-dose combinations. A practical approach is to prescribe two or more drugs sequentially with appropriate dose titrations of each; once blood pressure is controlled, an appropriate fixed-dose combination can be substituted. Alternatively, if at the start of therapy, multidrug treatment is believed to be necessary, a fixed-dose combination product can be prescribed. Currently, bisoprolol/hydrochlorothiazide (Ziac®) and captopril/hydrochlorothiazide (Capozide®) are the only fixed-dose combination products approved by the US Food and Drug Administration (FDA) for first-step therapy of hypertension. However, a number of effective fixed-dose combinations are available worldwide.

Why more fixed-dose combinations are not approved for first-step therapy in the United States relates to the regulatory position adopted by the FDA. According to the FDA, two or more drugs may be combined in a single dosage form when each component makes a contribution to the claimed effects. The dosage of each component should be such that the combination is safe and effective for a significant patient population requiring such concurrent therapy as defined in the drug labeling. The inherent excess risk of adverse effects caused by the addition of a second (or even a third) drug must be balanced by greater efficacy, the FDA states. The latter issue has proven a sticking point, and is the reason why fixed-dose combination drugs are not more widely approved in the United States as first-step therapy.

Fixed-dose combinations have not been studied as to cardiovascular outcomes, which is an additional consideration in their use as a first-step therapy. In that regard, the ACCOMPLISH study directly compared cardiovascular mortality and morbidity rates for two fixed-dose combination therapies—diuretic/ACE inhibitor and ACE inhibitor/CCB.

8. Can heart failure and renal disease be effectively treated with the amount of an ACE inhibitor or angiotensin-receptor antagonist (ARA) in a fixed-dose combination?

This is an interesting question, and one that is unlikely to be easily resolved. If fixed-dose combination therapy is employed as a means to affect blood-pressure reduction, then it may have a role in these disease states. But treatment with an ACE inhibitor or ARB in patients with heart failure requires careful upward dose titration to high amounts, which is not readily accomplished with a fixed-dose combination product. Moreover, the diuretic contained in all fixed-dose combination ACE inhibitor and ARB products is hydrochlorothiazide, which is not normally the preferred diuretic for the management of volume overload in the heart failure patient. Finally, in a negative sense, if fixed-dose combination therapy were considered in the heart failure patient as a way to reduce blood pressure, the health-care provider, because of its success in reducing blood pressure, might be dissuaded from the correct course of action, which is ACE inhibitor titration.

The current issues surrounding ACE inhibitor and ARB use in renal disease are still unresolved as to whether titration to treatment doses beyond those necessary for blood-pressure reduction should be routinely recommended for an additional antiproteinuric effect and/or renoprotection. Until the issue of dose titration in renal disease is more clearly defined, a fixed-dose combination product remains usable in the patient with renal disease (with or without proteinuria) when it can effectively reduce blood pressure. If dose titration of an ACE inhibitor or ARB to higher than currently recommended doses becomes the norm, then such dosage amounts would require that multiple pills of a particular product be taken. This could prove both cumbersome and possibly expose the patient to unnecessarily high amounts of the non-ACE inhibitor or non-ARB component of the combination.

9. Can fixed-dose combination therapy be used in patients with CKD and hypertension?

The role of pharmacokinetics and pharmacodynamics in response to fixed-dose combination products has been poorly described. For a number of fixed-dose combination products, their mode of action may be modified by the presence of comorbid conditions, eg, renal failure. A number of fixed-dose combination products contain an ACE inhibitor with either a diuretic or a CCB. In the case of the ACE inhibitor component of the fixed-dose combination, drug accumulation will begin as the glomerular filtration rate (GFR) falls below 60 mL/min. Any accumulation will then extend the duration of action of the ACE inhibitor component as well as the manner in which it interacts with either the accompanying diuretic or CCB. Available fixed-dose products that contain the ACE inhibitors trandolapril (ie, trandolapril/verapamil [Tarka®]) or fosinopril (fosinopril/hydrochlorothiazide [Monopril®-HCT]) would be the exceptions. Both of these ACE inhibitors use the hepatic route for at least 50% of their systemic clearance; thus, they are not subject to systemic accumulation with repetitive dosing in the setting of renal failure.

An additional consideration relates to the influence of the level of renal function on the action of the diuretic component of a fixed-dose combination product. It is believed that the early antihypertensive effect of a thiazide diuretic is governed by volume loss. Volume loss with thiazide diuretics depends on a number of factors, including the level of renal function. At a GFR <60 mL/min, the time of diuretic action will be modified, with varying effect, based upon the blood-pressure-lowering ability of a thiazide diuretic.

10. Is there a different dose-response relationship for the tissue-based effects of an antihypertensive compound than for its blood-pressure-lowering effect?

It is likely that different dose-response relationships exist for blood-pressure control and tissue protection, particularly for ACE inhibitors and ARBs. The nature of these dose-response relationships can only be speculated about at this time. Most fixed-dose combination products contain sufficient amounts of either an ACE inhibitor or ARB to reduce blood pressure, but presumably not enough of either compound to offer optimal tissue protection.

Until dosing recommendations specific to tissue protection are forthcoming, this is probably a moot point. More importantly, it should be remembered that the basis for the tissue protection we see with these compounds starts with an effective reduction in blood pressure. Fixed-dose combination therapy is usually more successful in reducing blood pressure than monotherapy with either an ACE inhibitor or ARB.

11. Are there disadvantages in using fixed-dose combination antihypertensive therapy?

A disadvantage in using fixed-dose combination antihypertensive therapy is a lack of dosing flexibility for its individual components. However, it is uncommon for physicians to maximally exploit the dosing flexibility inherent in the use of free combinations. With fixed-dose combination therapy, if additional amounts of either drug are required for blood-pressure control, a separate prescription may be required. This increases the complexity of the regimen and has the potential to negatively affect compliance. In addition, fixed-dose combination therapy may not provide adequate drug amounts to manage illnesses, ie, angina or heart failure, which commonly coexist with hypertension. As a result, β-blocker/diuretic fixed-dose combinations should not be recommended as primary therapy in the hypertensive patient with symptomatic CAD. Likewise, ACE inhibitor/diuretic and ACE inhibitor/CCB fixed-dose combinations provide inadequate amounts of ACE inhibitor for the effective treatment of systolic heart failure.

In addition, it has been suggested that fixed-dose combination antihypertensive therapy is pharmacokinetically irrational. This is a presumption based upon the differing half-lives for the individual components of the fixed-dose combination. This objection does not present an insurmountable hurdle to the use of fixed-dose combinations; rather, the opposite view can be taken that this is a therapeutic advantage. Too great a reduction in blood pressure may be avoided if the components of a combination product have differing times of peak effect. This is a valid consideration in the elderly where an excessive early hypotensive effect from multiple antihypertensive medications should be avoided.

Fixed-dose combination products should adhere to the therapeutic maxim for antihypertensive medications that a peak effect should be clinically tolerable with a major portion of the blood-pressure reduction sustained throughout the dosing interval. The duration of action of an antihypertensive agent frequently bears little relationship to its plasma half-life. A number of compounds given twice or three times daily as monotherapy (eg, β-blockers, ACE inhibitors) can be effective given once daily in a fixed-dose combination because of the potentiating effect of the coadministered compound.

Suggested Readings

Azor receives FDA approval for treatment of high blood pressure. *FDA Drug Approvals.* Available at: http://www.drugs.com/newdrugs/azor-receives-fda-approval-blood-pressure-655.html. Accessed September 11, 2008.

Bangalore S, Kamalakkannan G, Parkar S, et al: Fixed-dose combinations improve medication compliance: a meta-analysis. *Am J Med* 2007;120:713-719.

Exforge receives final US approval as new and powerful treatment option for patients with high blood pressure. *FDA Drug Approvals.* Available at: http://www.drugs.com/newdrugs/exforge-receives-final-us-approval-new-powerful-option-patients-blood-pressure-535.html. Accessed September 11, 2008.

Frishman WH, Bryzinski BS, Coulson LR, et al: A multifactorial trial design to assess combination therapy in hypertension. Treatment with bisoprolol and hydrochlorothiazide. *Arch Intern Med* 1994;154:1461-1468.

Jamerson KA, Bakris GL, Wun CC, et al: Rationale and design of the avoiding cardiovascular events through combination therapy in patients living with systolic hypertension (ACCOMPLISH) trial:

the first randomized controlled trial to compare the clinical outcome effects of first-line combination therapies in hypertension. *Am J Hypertens* 2004;17:793-801.

Law MR, Wald NJ, Morris JK, et al: Value of low dose combination treatment with blood pressure lowering drugs: analysis of 354 randomised trials. *BMJ* 2003;326:1427.

Neutel JM, Black HR, Weber MA: Combination therapy with diuretics: an evolution of understanding. *Am J Med* 1996;101:61S-70S.

Sever P: The heterogeneity of hypertension: why doesn't every patient respond to every antihypertensive drug? *J Hum Hypertens* 1995;9(suppl 2):S33-S36.

Sica DA: Rationale for fixed-dose combinations in the treatment of hypertension: the cycle repeats. *Drugs* 2002;62:443-462.

Waeber B: Very-low-dose combination: a first-line choice for the treatment of hypertension? *J Hypertens Suppl* 2003;21:S3-S10.

Weber MA, Ruilope L, Giles TD, et al: First-step use of fixed-dose combination treatment in stage 2 hypertensive patients: has the time come? *J Clin Hypertens (Greenwich)* 2007;9:276-284.

Weir MR: The rationale for combination versus single-entity therapy in hypertension. *Am J Hypertens* 1998;11:163S-169S.

Chapter 13

Special Populations

Over the past several decades, the United States has gained considerable ethnic diversity with hispanics representing 14% to 15% and blacks approximately 12% of the US population. Asians and Native Americans make up the remainder of the ethnic population. This phenomenon may be illustrated best by a review of the population demographic in California, which, according to the US Census Bureau, no longer has a majority population of nonhispanic whites. Obviously, if there is to be a meaningful impact on death and disability due to heart disease and stroke in the United States, the growing diversity of the US population needs to be more carefully considered.

High blood pressure is more common in ethnic and racial minority groups and the consequences of hypertension are more extreme in these groups, which is particularly the case in the black community. The frequency with which hypertension develops in blacks in the United States is high compared with hypertension rates for blacks in other areas of the world. In this regard, recent data demonstrate a gradient in risk across the African diaspora, with standardized hypertension prevalence rates of 14% in West Africa, and 26% in the Caribbean, compared with 33% in the United States. Of note, this geographic prevalence of hypertension matches a similar gradient in established risk factors, with obesity alone accounting for one third of the excess in hypertension found in the

United States compared with Africa. About 50% of the black population in the United States is located in the southeast. This is an important consideration because the prevalence of severe hypertension, as well as the risk of stroke and renal disease, is higher for blacks living in the southeast compared with blacks who live in other parts of the United States.

Target organ damage occurs with a disquieting frequency in blacks affected with hypertension. In blacks, end-stage renal disease (ESRD) is as much as 20-fold more likely to occur, both thrombotic and hemorrhagic stroke occur twice as often, and there is a 50% higher mortality from heart disease with left-ventricular hypertrophy (LVH) and heart failure occurring with a greater frequency than what is seen in whites. Currently, it is unclear in which order different antihypertensive therapies should be given to best improve cardiovascular outcomes in minority populations. In that regard, ethnicity is not a decisive factor in predicting the response to any class of antihypertensive therapy. Thus, there is virtually no justification to use ethnicity as the basis for avoiding selected drug classes because of an assumed lack of efficacy.

In most outcome trials, there is usually inadequate reporting of the number of minority participants. Most of the studies without race or ethnicity data were carried out in locations outside the United States (typically in the European Union), where trial reports are five times less likely to contain data on race or ethnicity than is the case for trials conducted in the United States. Race is particularly difficult to define in Latin American countries, given the considerable blending of indigenous peoples with those of European and/or African origin. Social, environmental, and lifestyle factors also differ greatly between hypertensive subjects in international trials and US minority subjects with shared geographic ancestry; these factors interact and may significantly influence cardiovascular risk and health outcomes.

Frequently Asked Questions

1. What pathobiological and clinical characteristics differentiate blacks with hypertension from whites with the disease?

Significant racial and ethnic diversity exists in the pathophysiology of essential hypertension, supporting the notion that this is a complex polygenetic disorder. The unique pathophysiologic and hemodynamic features of this condition in blacks must also be considered in the context of different mixes and intensities of supposed hypertension risk factors. That being said, compared with whites, blacks generally have a more volume-dependent, salt-sensitive form of hypertension in association with lower basal and/or stimulated levels of plasma-renin activity (PRA). Healthy normotensive young blacks also demonstrate impaired endothelial-dependent forearm vascular relaxation as measured by a decreased vasodilatory response to acetylcholine (ACh). This finding is similar to what has been observed in hypercholesterolemia, estrogen deficiency (ie, in post-menopausal women), aging, and/or hypertension.

Other neurohumoral abnormalities, ie, increased immunoreactive endothelin-I and transforming growth-factor β, and decreased levels of kallikrein-kinin, prostaglandin E_2, and atrial natriuretic peptide, have been observed in black hypertensives, although the cause and effect relationship between each and the onset and/or progression of hypertension is not well characterized. Not to be ignored in the black patient is the fact that socioeconomic factors (including access to health care), distrust of the health-care system, and late-stage disease diagnosis are significant modifiers of the course of hypertension.

2. Why do blacks have an increased prevalence of ESRD?

Hypertension is a major underlying cause of progressive chronic kidney disease (CKD) and continues to be a leading reason for the heavy burden of ESRD on blacks. Accordingly, the risk of incurring end-organ damage from hypertension differs in blacks, with the risk of developing ESRD several times higher than that observed in the white population. Late evaluation of black patients with CKD by a nephrologist occurs more often than not and is associated with a greater burden and severity of comorbid disease and a shorter duration of survival.

A number of explanations have been proffered to explain the persistently high rate of ESRD in blacks, a phenomenon which exists, although at a lower relative rate, even after controlling for differences in socioeconomic status and/or severity of blood pressure. Suggestions have included inadequate treatment of blood pressure; renal damage that is present before the initiation of therapy; familial clustering, albeit with a poorly worked out genetic pattern; birth weights <2,500 to 3,000 g; and/or the existence of intrinsic renal processes refractory to conventional therapy. As such, the kidneys of black and white hypertensives also exhibit important physiologic and pathologic differences. In this regard, black hypertensives typically exhibit much higher values for renal vascular resistance than do whites, which may relate to the production of much smaller amounts of the vasodilator bradykinin.

It has also been observed that daytime blood-pressure measurements may fail to capture the fact that blacks more frequently exhibit either higher nocturnal blood-pressure readings or a nondipping nocturnal blood-pressure pattern and that higher nocturnal blood pressure is not lowered with standard antihypertensive therapy. The racial findings related to nondipping nocturnal blood pressure are commonly found in American blacks but less so in non-American blacks. It is also probable that hypertensive renal injury is linked to salt sensitivity and insulin resistance, phenomena potentially exaggerated by a high dietary sodium intake.

3. What are important considerations in the nonpharmacologic management of hypertension in blacks?

The treatment of hypertension in black patients is a complex issue with overtones of socioeconomic status typically finding their way into the success or failure of any regimen. Blood-pressure screening remains an important tool in both prevention and effective management of hypertension and its sequelae in blacks. When coupled with risk factor modification counseling, screening programs offer the opportunity for meaningful intervention with respect to hypertension. There is also the issue of dietary intervention in the treatment of the black hypertensive. It is increasingly appreciated that the excess risk of hypertension in blacks may be due, in large measure, to a clustering of particular dietary inadequacies. The role of diet in blood-pressure control in the black hypertensive has frequently been studied. Recent studies employing the Dietary Approaches to Stop Hypertension (DASH) diet have provided a greater understanding of how certain dietary interventions affect a change in blood pressure. The DASH study was a randomized, controlled feeding study (459 adults with untreated systolic blood pressure <160 mm Hg and diastolic blood pressure of 80 to 95 mm Hg). Participants were provided with a normal 'control' diet for 3 weeks followed by randomization for 8 weeks to one of the following diets: (1) control diet; (2) a diet high in fruit and vegetable content; (3) a combination diet rich in fruits and vegetables and low-fat dietary foods, which had reduced levels of saturated fat, total fat, and cholesterol (ie, the DASH combination diet).

The DASH combination diet significantly lowered systolic and diastolic blood pressure. The fruits and vegetables diet similarly reduced blood pressure, but to a lesser extent than was seen with the DASH combination diet. The combination diet lowered systolic blood pressure significantly more in blacks (-6.8 mm Hg) than in whites

(-3 mm Hg) and in hypertensive subjects (-11.4 mm Hg) more than in nonhypertensive subjects (-3.4 mm Hg). The blood-pressure changes seen with the DASH combination diet occurred with weight and salt intake held constant. Thus, increased consumption of dairy products together with fruit and vegetables appears to be the preferred diet for reducing blood pressure and not one simply emphasizing decreased salt intake. At the very least, if a DASH diet cannot be put into practice, dietary potassium and calcium can be increased, in concert with a plan to reduce body weight and decrease stress levels.

4. What is the response to various antihypertensive medication classes in blacks?

It has been well documented that, as monotherapy or in the absence of diuretic therapy, β-blockers, angiotensin-converting enzyme (ACE) inhibitors, and angiotensin-receptor blockers (ARBs) do not lower blood pressure to the same extent in black patients as they do in white patients with hypertension. It has also been observed that thiazide diuretics and calcium-channel blockers (CCBs) have greater blood-pressure-lowering efficacy in blacks than do other drug classes. With the above observations in mind, several additional therapeutic maxims deserve comment.

First, multidrug therapy is more often than not required in blacks, with a diuretic as an important component of any such regimen. Additional consideration also should be given in this population to the use of aldosterone-receptor antagonists (ARAs) and combined α-/β-blockers. Second, although β-blockers, ACE inhibitors, and ARBs do not lower blood pressure to the same extent in black patients as in white patients, in a portion of the black population they do lower blood pressure effectively; therefore, it cannot be assumed that these drug classes would not be effective in individual black patients. Finally, the perception that it is uniformly more difficult to lower blood pressure in a black patient than in other patients is unfounded. If careful attention is directed toward combining antihypertensive drug classes, blood pressure can be effectively controlled even in black patients with hypertension and moderate-to-advanced CKD.

5. What are important considerations in South Asians with hypertension?

Hypertension and cardiovascular disease (CVD) (Indian Asians account for one fifth of all cardiovascular deaths worldwide) are major public health problems in the Indian subcontinent and among South Asians worldwide. Although the prevalence of hypertension is lower in rural (compared with urban) Indian populations, there has been a continuous increase in hypertension prevalence in both settings. The emigration effects on hypertension prevalence, although somewhat variable, would suggest that psychosocial and nutritional variables (ie, genetic/environmental interaction) unique to the region of emigration determine the expression of the hypertensive state. A decidedly more common finding relating to emigration has been the high rate of CVD among expatriate Indians no matter where they emigrate.

Several possibilities exist for the increasing prevalence of hypertension in South Asians—acculturation and urbanization of the population, excessive tobacco use in diverse and smokeless forms, an increase in fat and oil consumption, and a population becoming ever more obese. A high rate of diabetes, central obesity, and other features of the metabolic syndrome (especially the characteristic dyslipidemia of reduced high-density lipoprotein cholesterol [HDL-C] and raised triglycerides [Tgs]) have also been reported in migrant and urban Indian populations. However, there is limited data on the detection, treatment, and control of hypertension in the Asian-Indian population. Asian-Indian ethnicity also appears not to define the response pattern to antihypertensive medication classes. However, it would be expected that the obesity present in this population would make it a more salt-sensitive population.

As such, diuretics and CCBs might be expected to be the most effective in reducing blood pressure in South Asians.

6. What are important considerations in Native Americans related to hypertension and end-organ disease?

Striking heterogeneity among the more than 500 Native-American tribes in the United States along with geographic dispersion and both cultural and language barriers have made the accumulation of data on Native Americans a challenge. In the past, the rates of risk factors for atherosclerosis and CVD as well as the manifestations of coronary heart disease (CHD), stroke, and peripheral vascular disease (PVD) in Native Americans have been low compared with the general US population. However, over the past several decades, the rates of these CVD-associated risk factors have noticeably increased in Native Americans with a not insignificant accompanying rise in the manifestations of atherosclerosis.

As a result, CVD is now the leading cause of death in Native Americans, and hypertension is a strong predictor for the development of diabetes-associated complications, ie, retinopathy, renal disease. Recent longitudinal population surveys on Native Americans show that the risk of developing hypertension is on the rise, that the incidence of hypertension is high, and that systolic forms of hypertension predominate. Moreover, prehypertensive Native Americans have three times the risk of developing hypertension and almost twice the risk of developing CVD as do normotensives.

Native Americans and Alaska natives have high rates of CKD, in both diabetics and nondiabetics. Although Native Americans comprise just 1.5% of the US population, they have the highest rate of diabetes in the world and also one of the highest rates of ESRD. The rate of ESRD among Native Americans with diabetes is about sixfold higher than what is observed in non-Native Americans. There is also significant regional variation as well as differences among the approximately 550 tribes that comprise the Native-American community, with certain tribes having ESRD rates >20 times those of whites.

7. *What is the response to various antihypertensive medication classes in hispanics?*

Patient racial, ethnic, and socioeconomic characteristics can affect health-care access, and hispanics are less likely to have a regular health-care provider and health insurance than are blacks or whites. Interventions aimed at improving blood-pressure control rates in hispanics may be especially important due to the growth in this population segment. While hispanics comprised 12.6% of the US population in 2000, census data estimate that, by 2050, almost 25% of the US population will be hispanic. Although there are few published studies of drug efficacy in hispanics, there appears to be no hierarchy in response to the various antihypertensive drug classes. Blood-pressure control can be achieved with commonly available medications, and hispanic ethnicity is not associated with inferior control in the clinical trial setting (ie, the Antihypertensive and Lipid-Lowering Treatment to Prevent Heart Attack Trial [ALLHAT]) in which hypertensive patients had equal access to medical care and medication was provided at no cost.

Suggested Readings

Brewster LM, van Montfrans GA, Kleijnen J: Systematic review: antihypertensive drug therapy in black patients. *Ann Intern Med* 2004;141:614-627.

Drukteinis JS, Roman MJ, Fabsitz RR, et al: Cardiac and systemic hemodynamic characteristics of hypertension and prehypertension in adolescents and young adults: the Strong Heart Study. *Circulation* 2007;115:221-227.

Ferdinand KC: Hypertension in minority populations. *J Clin Hypertens (Greenwich)* 2006;8:365-368.

Giles T, Aranda JM Jr, Suh DC, et al: Ethnic/racial variations in blood pressure awareness, treatment, and control. *J Clin Hypertens (Greenwich)* 2007;9:345-354.

Jamerson K, DeQuattro V: The impact of ethnicity on response to antihypertensive therapy. *Am J Med* 1996;101:22S-32S.

Margolis KL, Piller LB, Ford CE, et al: Blood pressure control in Hispanics in the antihypertensive and lipid-lowering treatment to prevent heart attack trial. *Hypertension* 2007;50:854-861.

Narva AS: The spectrum of kidney disease in American Indians. *Kidney Int Suppl* 2003;83:S3-S7.

Park IU, Taylor AL: Race and ethnicity in trials of antihypertensive therapy to prevent cardiovascular outcomes: a systematic review. *Ann Fam Med* 2007;5:444-452.

Srinath Reddy K, Shah B, Varghese C, et al: Responding to the threat of chronic diseases in India. *Lancet* 2005;366:1744-1749.

Yeates K, Tonelli M: Indigenous health: update on the impact of diabetes and chronic kidney disease. *Curr Opin Nephrol Hypertens* 2006;15:588-592.

Chapter 14

Treatment of Hypertension in the Athlete and the Exercising Patient

The importance of exercise as a part of a lifestyle modification plan to control blood pressure and to reduce the likelihood of cardiovascular events has been well described in the literature. Cardiovascular disease (CVD) increases with age, and, at every age, there is a continuous relationship between blood-pressure levels and cardiovascular events. Increases in blood pressure are common with stress, exercise, and anger. Consequently, it is of interest to know whether we are putting our older patients at risk for cardiovascular events by recommending aerobic exercise, particularly if they are not well conditioned. Much still needs to be learned about how to safely intensify exercise regimens and how to interpret blood pressure and heart responses during exercise.

Frequently Asked Questions

1. Does the rise in blood pressure during exercise increase the risk for cardiovascular events? How much of a blood pressure rise is too much?

The rise in blood pressure associated with exercise treadmill testing (ETT) may provide clinical clues as to the risk for cardiovascular events. Some clinicians have suggested that a prolonged period before returning to a baseline blood pressure may predict those individuals at an increased risk of cardiovascular events. Some clinical investigation also suggests that systolic blood pressures >200 mm Hg during peak exercise may be indicative of a patient who has CVD and is at increased risk for cardiovascular events. Others have suggested that an increase in systolic blood pressure of >60 mm Hg from a resting blood-pressure measurement is also indicative of CVD and increased cardiovascular risk. Others have suggested that exaggerated rises of blood pressure during exercise identifies patients with fixed hypertension. Left-ventricular hypertrophy (LVH) is also associated with peak systolic blood pressures >200 mm Hg during exercise.

2. Should older exercising patients receive ETT to evaluate whether there may be clinically relevant coronary disease and to assess their blood-pressure responses during the course of exercise should patients receive antihypertensive medication to blunt the increase in blood pressure observed during exercise?

This is a question that is difficult to answer, given that there is insufficient literature to evaluate changes in blood pressure during exercise and the resultant risk for cardiovascular events, and whether treatment will reduce this risk. It still has not been definitively proven whether patients would benefit from medication to minimize exercise-induced changes in blood pressure.

3. Which drugs would best facilitate control of blood pressure during exercise, yet not interfere with exercise-induced changes in heart rate and stroke volume?

Exercise-induced changes in blood pressure that remain abnormal during the course of exercise may indicate patients who have masked hypertension. This is a disease entity in which blood pressures are within the normal range during office visits at rest, but, when measured with ambulatory blood-pressure monitoring techniques, are abnormal during the course of daily living, whether at work, during exercise, or in other activities of daily living. Masked hypertension may also reflect the response to a stressful job or living environment, and it does correlate with increased surrogate measures of CVD and coronary artery disease (CAD) risk. Consequently, abnormal blood-pressure patterns during exercise may be helpful in identifying patients at risk for CAD and in whom antihypertensive therapy would be indicated.

Although not well studied, it is reasonable to suggest that all major forms of blood-pressure-lowering therapy could be used in the exercising patient. However, caution should be used with β-blockers. These agents would need to be titrated carefully to allow sufficient heart-rate response during exercise so that there would be no compromise in stroke volume. This is particularly an issue in a patient who is initiating an exercise program and in whom necessary heart-rate responses are important, given their poor level of conditioning. Even in conditioned athletes with low resting heart rates, further reduction in heart rate could impair exercise tolerance by inducing fatigue.

Nondihydropyridine calcium-channel blockers (NCCBs), ie, verapamil (Calan®, Covera-HS®, Isoptin® SR, Verelan®) or diltiazem (Cardizem®, Cartia®, Dilacor® XR, Diltia®, Diltzac®, Tiazac®), which have modest negative chronotrophic effects, but more predominate peripheral vasodilatory effects, may be more suitable in the individual who wishes to undertake an exercise program. Modest reduction of heart rate coupled with peripheral vasodilatation may be the ideal means of controlling blood pressure during the course of exercise and limiting the sensation of fatigue. Other vasodilators, ie, ACE inhibitors, angiotensin-receptor blockers (ARBs), may also be employed, and, if there are considerations of mild volume excess, low doses of thiazide diuretics also could be prescribed.

More clinical trials are needed to evaluate the advantages and disadvantages of different therapeutic strategies in the exercising patient and to also address the issue of just how much systolic and diastolic blood-pressure control is optimal.

4. Should hypertensive patients be encouraged to begin exercise programs?

We should continue to encourage hypertensive patients to exercise as a means to control weight, to facilitate physical conditioning, and to reduce the likelihood of CVD progression. However, each exercise program needs to be initiated in a cautious and sensible manner to avoid overstressing the patient's circulation. This is particularly important in hypertensive patients who are poorly conditioned. It may also be an important consideration in older patients who have abnormal blood-pressure responses to exercise and in whom peak changes in blood pressure could lead to vascular events.

5. Does the delayed fall in systolic blood pressure postexercise indicate CVD and an increased risk for cardiovascular events? Is the fall in blood pressure during exercise worrisome?

A delayed fall in blood pressure postexercise could indicate that a patient has CVD and abnormal endogenous vasorelaxation responses, which may reflect a damaged endothelium with impaired nitric oxide (NO) production or responsiveness. However, it also could indicate excess oxidative stress from the blood-pressure rise, which could overwhelm endogenous vasodilatory responses. Some investigators have suggested that blood pressure should fall to baseline pre-exercise levels within 5 minutes after completion of exercise. In patients with systolic heart failure, the decrement of blood pressure during exercise is considered an adverse prognostic sign for cardiovascular events.

6. Is there also a decrement in blood pressure in the exercising patient who does not show any evidence of systolic heart failure?

The answer to this question may be of particular interest in patients who have a longstanding history of hypertension and LVH associated with some degree of diastolic dysfunction. In this patient, increased heart rate during exercise could conceivably compromise LV filling during diastole and result in a fall in cardiac output.

7. Could antioxidant therapy or NO stimulating therapies help overcome excessive exercise-mediated increases in blood pressure?

Possibly yes. This is a fertile area of clinical research. Drugs that block the RAAS or direct NO stimulating therapies also are of some interest. Because of its antioxidant effects, vitamin C also is being studied.

Suggested Readings

Abe K, Tsuda M, Hayashi H, et al: Diagnostic usefulness of post-exercise systolic blood pressure response for detection of coronary artery disease in patients with electrocardiographic left ventricular hypertrophy. *Am J Cardiol* 1995;76:892-895.

Acanfora D, De Caprio L, Cuomo S, et al: Diagnostic value of the ratio of recovery systolic blood pressure to peak exercise systolic blood pressure for the detection of coronary artery disease. *Circulation* 1988;77:1306-1310.

Ajisaka R, Watanabe S, Masuoka T, et al: The significance of abnormal systolic blood pressure response during supine ergometer exercise and postexercise in ischemic heart disease, studied by exercise radionuclide ventriculography. *Jpn Heart J* 1989;30:163-179.

Allison TG, Cordeiro MA, Miller TD, et al: Prognostic significance of exercise-induced systemic hypertension in healthy subjects. *Am J Cardiol* 1999;83:371-375.

Amon KW, Richards KL, Crawford MH: Usefulness of the post-exercise response of systolic blood pressure in the diagnosis of coronary artery disease. *Circulation* 1984;70:951-956.

Fletcher GF, Balady GJ, Amsterdam EA, et al: Exercise standards for testing and training: a statement for healthcare professionals from the American Heart Association. *Circulation* 2001;104:1694-1740.

Goel R, Majeed F, Vogel R, et al: Exercise-induced hypertension, endothelial dysfunction, and coronary artery disease in a marathon runner. *Am J Cardiol* 2007;99:743-744.

Jurva JW, Phillips SA, Syed AQ, et al: The effect of exertional hypertension evoked by weight lifting on vascular endothelial function. *J Am Coll Cardiol* 2006;48:588-589.

Stewart KJ, Ouyang P, Bacher AC, et al: Exercise effects on cardiac size and left ventricular diastolic function: relationships to changes in fitness, fatness, blood pressure and insulin resistance. *Heart* 2006;92:893-898.

Syme AN, Blanchard BE, Guidry MA, et al: Peak systolic blood pressure on a graded maximal exercise test and the blood pressure response to an acute bout of submaximal exercise. *Am J Cardiol* 2006;98:938-943.

Taylor AJ, Beller GA: Postexercise systolic blood pressure response: association with the presence and extent of perfusion abnormalities on thallium-201 scintigraphy. *Am Heart J* 1995;129:227-234.

Tsuda M, Hatano K, Hayashi H, et al: Diagnostic value of post-exercise systolic blood pressure response for detecting coronary artery disease in patients with or without hypertension. *Am Heart J* 1993;125:718-725.

Chapter 15

Salt Intake, Nonsteroidal Anti-Inflammatory Drugs, and Hypertension

The Western diet is replete with salt. Although there has been much debate in the literature concerning the relationship between dietary salt and blood pressure, there certainly is no evidence to indicate that dietary salt deficiency exists in modern societies of the developed world. If anything, there is more concern that, with an aging population and increased obesity, these susceptible population groups may experience more problems with salt-related increases in blood pressure.

Nonsteroidal anti-inflammatory drugs (NSAIDs) possess both anti-inflammatory and analgesic properties that make NSAIDs a useful therapeutic strategy for many patients with acute or chronic pain, or inflammatory syndromes. Consequently, NSAIDs are some of the most commonly prescribed medications in the world. In addition, in many countries, they are available in over-the-counter preparations.

What many patients do not appreciate is that NSAIDs have antinatriuretic effects and can induce dose-dependent salt and water retention, which can result in an increase in blood pressure. The interesting question is how much blood-pressure change is expected in a given patient, and what is the relationship of that change with the patient's concomitant dietary salt intake?

Most clinical studies that have employed detailed measures of salt ingestion and excretion have demonstrated consistent increases in fluid retention and blood pressure with NSAIDs. This is more pronounced in patients with a higher salt intake, given the antinatriuretic effects of these drugs. On average, the increase in systolic blood pressure in NSAID users is 4 to 5 mm Hg. In addition, the change in blood-pressure response to NSAID use is magnified in patients who are older and in those with hypertension, heart disease, or renal disease. Few studies have been conducted to evaluate the effect on blood pressure of NSAIDs in people with hypertension.

Frequently Asked Questions

1. How much salt is too much to ingest when taking NSAIDs?

Since NSAIDs are chemicals that have antinatriuretic effects, their impact on plasma volume and pressure is directly proportional to dietary salt consumption. With more salt ingestion, there is a greater net effect on blood pressure. However, the net effect on blood pressure may also depend on the patient's current blood-pressure level, the presence or absence of chronic kidney disease (CKD), concomitant medications for blood pressure, and perhaps other dietary factors. In general, a patient on chronic NSAID therapy should reduce his or her dietary salt consumption.

2. Are there differences between NSAIDs and their risk of causing higher levels of blood pressure?

There is a marked heterogeneity of blood-pressure responses in clinical trials that have been performed to evaluate different types of NSAID therapy. Often, casual blood-pressure readings are used, which may not be entirely reflective of the net effect of different types of NSAIDs on blood pressure. However, it has been quite consistent that whether one is using a traditional NSAID that inhibits both isoforms of cyclooxygenase (ie, COX 1, COX 2) or the newer COX 1-selective NSAIDs, the overall effect on blood pressure is almost identical. This effect can be explained by the similar action of traditional NSAIDs and coxibs on the handling of sodium and water by the kidneys. COX 2 is the dominant regulator of prostaglandin production in the macula densa and renal medullary interstitium, which are the principal areas involved in the regulation of sodium and water by the kidneys. It is not surprising that both traditional NSAIDs and coxibs have similar effects on blood pressure. Another important issue may be the duration of action of these different drugs. The longer the duration of action, the greater the effect, whereas the shorter duration of action, the less the effect. Thus, the longer-acting drugs would have a more profound effect on the retention of salt and water and on blood pressure, whereas the shorter-acting drugs would have less of an effect.

3. Does the dose of NSAID make a difference in the change in blood pressure?

It is quite likely that the dose of NSAID, whether it is a traditional COX 1 and COX 2 blocker or newer COX 2-selective blocker, has an effect on salt and water retention. As the effects of COX inhibition appear to be dose dependent, the higher the dose of drug, the greater the impact on salt and water retention. It is preferable to always use the lowest possible dose of NSAID to achieve the desired anti-inflammatory or analgesic effect to avoid a more pronounced effect on salt and water retention.

4. What is the best way to monitor the effect of NSAIDs on blood volume and pressure?

When requiring chronic NSAID therapy, all patients should be advised to weigh themselves every day. They should also modify their dietary salt intake and evaluate their blood pressure with a home blood-pressure-measuring device. Clinical studies show that one week of chronic daily NSAID use often will result in the retention of about 150 mEq of sodium. This is analogous to about 1 L of saline and would cause an expected increase in weight of approximately 2 lbs. The net impact of this change in weight often results in a change in blood pressure of about 4 to 5 mm Hg. However, the expected change in blood pressure in a given patient can vary substantially, depending upon the level of pretreatment blood pressure, the presence of renal disease, other dietary factors, and concomitant medications. For those patients with higher levels of blood pressure, more careful monitoring is in order. Patients with an estimated glomerular filtration rate (eGFR) <60 mL/min/1.73 m^2 should also be closely monitored. Because some NSAIDs are available over the counter, they may be used indiscriminately by patients who do not realize that they are at a higher risk for renal disease or hypertension and could also increase their risk for more substantial changes in blood pressure.

5. What is the best way to reduce the dose of NSAIDs to minimize their effect on blood pressure?

This is an important question, which is difficult to answer in a general way. Often one needs to start with a higher dose of an NSAID to treat acute pain. However, one can titrate to lower doses as the symptoms abate and can then space out the dose to create a longer 'off' period so that there is a lesser effect on the kidneys. Sometimes switching from a longer-acting NSAID to a shorter-acting NSAID can help. It may also be advisable to supplement the patient with acetaminophen or perhaps a low dose of an opiate to reduce the need for the analgesic requirements of an NSAID, yet maintain a sufficient dose of the drug for its anti-inflammatory effect. These approaches need to be carefully individualized to maintain symptom control and to minimize the risk of changes in blood pressure.

6. What are the most effective drugs to use for blood-pressure control in the patient who requires chronic NSAID therapy?

Calcium-channel blockers (CCBs) are the one form of antihypertensive therapy that may provide the most robust ability to control blood pressure even during chronic NSAID use. This effect has been demonstrated in a number of clinical trials, and it may be related to the intrinsic natriuretic properties of CCBs, which are likely not dependent on prostaglandin production. This is in contradiction to diuretics, particularly loop-acting drugs, which are susceptible to the effects of NSAIDs. β-Blockers and drugs that block the renin-angiotensin-aldosterone system (RAAS) (ie, angiotensin-converting enzyme [ACE] inhibitors, angiotensin-receptor blockers [ARBs]) are also susceptible to the hypertensive effects of NSAIDs. Clinical studies have also demonstrated that β-blockers and RAAS blocking drugs are less effective in lowering blood pressure in volume-replete individuals. Regardless of the types of medications in the antihypertensive regimen, whenever chronic NSAID therapy is introduced, patients need to be monitored carefully for changes in blood pressure and appropriate medication modifications should be made during the course of treatment.

One other concern with chronic NSAID therapy is in patients who receive drugs that block the RAAS. Both NSAIDs and RAAS blockers interfere with potassium excretion, and substantial increases in serum-potassium levels may occur with concomitant use of these drugs. As a result, serum-potassium levels should be monitored carefully, especially in patients with eGFR <60 mL/min/1.73 m^2 Patients should also be advised not to use salt substitutes, as these products also contain potassium and may result in substantial increases in serum-potassium levels.

Suggested Readings

Brater DC: Effects of nonsteroidal anti-inflammatory drugs on renal function: focus on cyclooxygenase-2-selective inhibition. *Am J Med* 1999;107:65S-70S.

DeMaria AN, Weir MR: Coxibs--beyond the GI tract: renal and cardiovascular issues. *J Pain Symptom Manage* 2003;25(2 suppl): S41-S49.

Salzberg DJ, Weir MR: COX-2 inhibitors and cardiovascular risk. *Subcell Biochem* 2007;42:159-174.

Weir MR: Microalbuminuria and cardiovascular disease. *Clin J Am Soc Nephrol* 2007;2:581-590.

Weir MR: Salt intake and hypertensive renal injury in African-Americans. A therapeutic perspective. *Am J Hypertens* 1995;8: 635-644.

Weir MR, Sperling RS, Reicin A, et al: Selective COX-2 inhibition and cardiovascular effects: a review of the rofecoxib development program. *Am Heart J* 2003;146:591-604.

Chapter **16**

Drug-Resistant Hypertension

Before embarking on a patient work-up for secondary hypertension, the clinician should establish that the medication regimen used has not produced pseudotolerance and/or that the prescribed regimen is being taken. Pseudotolerance derives from counterregulatory responses, ie, tachycardia, plasma-volume expansion, renin-angiotensin-aldosterone system (RAAS)/sympathetic nervous system (SNS) activation, that are sufficiently operational to blunt the blood-pressure-lowering effect of antihypertensive medications. When pseudotolerance develops, it most commonly relates to unrecognized plasma-volume expansion, which can occur with several antihypertensive classes including centrally acting agents, β-blockers, and/or direct vasodilators, ie, hydralazine, minoxidil. The salt and water retention with minoxidil can be particularly prominent and a major factor behind the occasional loss of effect of this compound.

It is poorly appreciated as to how small an increase in plasma volume (peripheral edema is frequently absent) can significantly increase blood pressure. This process can take place even during ongoing diuretic therapy and is particularly common when there is a significant divergence between dietary sodium intake and the natriuretic response to the administered diuretic. Reducing plasma volume, either with an increase in the dose of an existing diuretic or by conversion to a more potent diuretic, can appreciably reduce blood pressure in many patients with resistant hypertension.

Another form of pseudoresistance surfaces when the RAAS is activated, which may occur with high-dose diuretic and/or nonspecific vasodilator therapy (ie, hydralazine, minoxidil). Such a possibility can be tested with random sampling for plasma-renin activity (PRA) and plasma-aldosterone (PA) concentrations. In the course of such testing, the patient should be in an upright position, and, whenever possible, should have been without antihypertensive medications for 8 to 12 hours. In most cases, PRA values 73 ng/mL/hr represent excess angiotensin II (Ang II) effect and the likelihood that drugs that cut back activity in this system, ie, angiotensin-converting enzyme (ACE) inhibitors, angiotensin-receptor blockers (ARBs), will further reduce blood pressure. PA values >10 ng/dL usually represent an excess of this neurohormone and are also an indicator that aldosterone should be a specific therapeutic target. Contrary to popular belief, chronic ACE inhibitor and ARB therapy does not reduce PA values; thus, if a reduction in aldosterone effect is desired, an aldosterone-receptor antagonist (ARA), ie, eplerenone (Inspra®), spironolactone (Aldactone®), is required.

Frequently Asked Questions

1. What is a reasonable working definition for resistant hypertension?

Resistant hypertension is generally defined as the failure to attain goal blood pressure in adherent patients despite three maximally titrated medications when one of those medications is a diuretic. Resistant hypertension can occur in a primary fashion, if the desired blood pressure is never reached, or in a secondary manner, if blood-pressure control lapses after having been originally well controlled. The latter situation is commonly due to drug-related counter-regulatory responses or pseudotolerance. The existence of resistant hypertension can serve as a clue to the presence of a secondary form of hypertension, but, more often, it is a reflection of a physician's treatment attitudes and goals, medication nonadherence, or pathophysiologic problems, ie, sleep disorders, anxiety, and/or depression, As a result, resistant hypertension is often not resistant per se; rather it can simply be an indicator of inadequately treated hypertension as may occur with the dose and types of medications chosen.

2. Is noncompliance a common cause of apparent drug-resistant hypertension?

It cannot be overstated how important it is to establish medication compliance before embarking on a diagnostic work-up for a secondary cause of hypertension. A carefully documented patient history, discussions with family members (or significant others), or checking pharmacy refill records can prove useful in establishing poor compliance as the basis for resistant hypertension. Physical examination clues can also occasionally provide an indication of medication use (or not), particularly when high medication doses are being given. The lack of reflex tachycardia or hair growth in a minoxidil-treated patient, the absence of a heart-rate reduction (or bradycardia) in a β-blocker-treated patient, a calcium-channel-blocker (CCB)-treated patient lacking peripheral edema or a clonidine (Catapres®)-treated patient without dry mouth or sedation can be indicators of possible medication noncompliance.

Another consideration in apparent drug-resistant hypertension is measurement error. A common measurement error takes place when a cuff is used that is too small for the arm, and the blood pressure is systematically overestimated. In general, the cuff should be large enough for the bladder to encircle at least 75% of the upper arm circumference and to extend at least two thirds of its length. Pseudohypertension is an uncommon cause of resistant hypertension and is due to the noncompressibility of severely atherosclerotic or calcified brachial or radial arteries. This condition should be suspected when hypotension symptoms regularly arise without a change in blood pressure (by cuff measurement). Direct intra-arterial blood-pressure measurement is usually needed to prove the presence of this condition.

3. How often is white-coat hypertension the cause of resistant hypertension?

Blood pressure at rest does not predict the response an individual may manifest during physical or emotional stress. About 20% of patients with office blood-pressure readings not at goal do not have hypertension on home or ambulatory blood-pressure monitoring, which is a phenomenon termed the white-coat effect or white-coat hypertension. Of note, office blood pressure is poorly responsive to usual antihypertensive medications in the patient with white-coat hypertension. At the same time, white-coat hypertensives may exhibit an excessive response to medications at home. Patients with white-coat hypertension also often discontinue medications and can present considerable management problems to the clinician until a correct diagnosis is made.

The issue often arises as to the validity of home readings that differ substantially from those obtained in the office setting. If the home readings are in dispute, then one way to qualify such readings is to look for the presence of significant or progressive target-organ damage. In that regard, an echocardiogram looking for evidence of left-ventricular hypertrophy (LVH) can prove helpful. Although white-coat hypertension was initially thought to be transient and, therefore, benign, there is now increasing evidence to suggest that the prognosis for white-coat hypertensives falls at least midway between that for those with normotension and established hypertension.

A final consideration is that a group of patients exist that have been variously labeled with the terms reverse white-coat hypertension and white-coat normotension or more recently masked hypertension. Such patients resemble true hypertensive patients in all aspects other than having normal clinic blood-pressure readings. This is in contrast to readings in the home or work environment, which are in the hypertensive range. Recent studies have shown that patients with masked hypertension are at higher risk than those with responder hypertension. Because office blood-pressure measurements do not recognize individuals with masked hypertension, ambulatory blood-pressure monitoring is required to make this diagnosis.

4. How is plasma-volume expansion best managed in the patient with resistant hypertension?

Clinically, it is often difficult to gauge the extent to which counterregulatory systems are activated in the treated hypertensive patient, although a fairly reliable sign is an unexplained loss of existing blood-pressure control. Salt retention, as a means by which blood-pressure control is lost, is easy to recognize if peripheral edema develops, but salt retention as a factor in loss of blood-pressure control can still (and often does) occur without peripheral edema. If the latter is suspected, a diuretic can be started (or if one is already in use, its dose can be increased) to affect a small weight loss.

What constitutes a small weight loss is patient dependent in the individual with resistant hypertension. If a patient is edematous, then resolution of the edema state and/or normalization of blood pressure can be used as benchmarks for the desired response to an adjusted diuretic regimen. In the nonedematous patient, a 2% to 3% reduction in body weight generally is sufficient to establish whether a recent lapse in blood-pressure control has been the result of plasma-volume expansion.

Adjusting diuretic therapy in the resistant hypertensive with suspected plasma-volume expansion should occur in a fairly systematic manner. First, because hydrochlorothiazide (Esidrix®, Microzide®) is the most commonly used diuretic, its dose can be increased (maximum=50 mg) and the response assessed. This maneuver is typically of limited utility in that hydrochlorothiazide is a fairly weak and short-acting diuretic. Switching from hydrochlorothiazide to the more long-acting, thiazide diuretic chlorthalidone is the preferred first course of action. Patients prescribed chlorthalidone often lose weight, and, in addition, chlorthalidone also is more effective at lowering blood pressure than hydrochlorothiazide.

Finally, if circumstances dictate (presence of significant renal failure or heavy proteinuria), a switch can be made from a thiazide diuretic to a loop diuretic. In so doing, if furosemide (Lasix®) (a short-acting compound) is used, twice-daily dosing is often necessary; alternatively, the loop diuretic torsemide (Demadex®) can be given once daily due to its longer half-life. The occasional patient (minoxidil-treated and/or one with nephrotic syndrome) requires combination therapy with a loop and a thiazide diuretic (ie, metolazone [Zaroxolyn®]) for maintenance of fluid balance.

5. What drugs are commonly linked to hypertension?

A number of drugs are associated with new-onset (or worsening of pre-existing) hypertension. Any medication (or ingested substance) causing hypertension does so through specific mechanisms—there are compounds that cause salt and water retention, there are substances that activate the SNS (and occasionally the RAAS), and there are medications and/or substances that specifically alter vascular structure and function and, in so doing, elevate blood pressure by raising peripheral resistance. A careful inventory of medications and ingested substances is critical in the patient with resistant hypertension because potentially offending agents should be identified early in the course of therapy.

Synthetic corticosteroids dose dependently increase blood pressure in about 20% of patients who receive these compounds. This form of hypertension is typically characterized by plasma-volume expansion and is best managed by tapering (or discontinuing) the steroid; however, if this is not possible, then diuretic or CCB therapy may be used with adjunct sympatholytic therapy as needed. Oral contraceptives induce hypertension in about 5% of users of high-dose compounds containing at least 50 μg of estrogen and 1 to 4 mg of progestin. Increases in blood pressure, albeit within the normal range, are also common in women who use birth control pills. Oral contraceptives produce changes in the RAAS, particularly a consistent marked increase in the plasma-renin substrate concentration, which may be associated with increases in PRA and aldosterone excretion. The hypertension seen in women using oral contraceptives typically remits upon discontinuation of the therapy, but it may sometimes be weeks or even months before blood-pressure levels return to baseline value. In the interim, agents that block the RAAS and/or ARAs (with or without a diuretic) may be helpful in controlling blood pressure.

Nonsteroidal anti-inflammatory drugs (NSAIDs) can increase blood pressure. This rise in blood pressure is most commonly seen in the elderly, those with pre-existing hypertension, salt-sensitive hypertensives, or patients with chronic kidney disease (CKD). NSAIDs also blunt the blood-pressure-lowering effect of all antihypertensive medication classes other than CCBs. Individual NSAIDs may differ somewhat in their capacity to increase blood pressure, primarily relating to potency and half-life. Either acute or chronic use of excessive amounts of alcohol is another common cause of hypertension and often is the basis for resistant hypertension. In certain instances, blood-pressure control is impossible unless there is complete abstinence from alcohol. Failure on the part of a patient to divulge their true level of alcohol intake should always be a consideration in the patient with resistant hypertension.

Drugs that affect sympathetic neurotransmission can often increase blood pressure, eg, phenylephrine, cocaine. Combination α-/β-blocker medications are useful therapies for this form of hypertension, which is typically more acute than chronic in nature. Antiobesity drugs (ie, sibutramine [Meridia®]) and numerous neuropsychiatric medications can increase blood pressure. In the case of neuropsychiatric medications, the underlying psychiatric disorder needs to be considered as a potential contributor to the blood-pressure pattern. As such, panic disorders or so-called 'panic blood-pressure physiology' is not uncommon. Finally, recombinant erythropoietin can be associated with the onset of hypertension anywhere from weeks to months after beginning therapy. Tempering the rate (and absolute hemoglobin value attained) of blood-pressure rise lessens the risk of developing significant hypertension. Once present, however, multiple medications are usually required because this form of hypertension can prove quite difficult to control.

6. Can a pheochromocytoma be a cause of resistant hypertension?

The predominant secretory pattern for catecholamines (ie, epinephrine, norepinephrine, and/or other neurohormones) influences the symptom profile of a pheochromocytoma. Symptoms, including a pattern of blood-pressure elevation, do not necessarily correlate with the size of a tumor. The triad of symptoms that typify pheochromocytoma is headaches, excessive/generalized sweating, and palpitations; however, the symptom pattern of a pheochromocytoma can be quite varied with other common symptoms including pallor, weight loss, and feelings of panic and anxiety. Most (but not all) of the clinical signs and symptoms of a pheochromocytoma are due to the direct actions of secreted catecholamines.

There is not a specific blood-pressure pattern that is absolutely pathognomic for a pheochromocytoma. The blood-pressure patterns seen with a pheochromocytoma include a sustained hypertensive state with no volatility, a persistent hypertensive state with occasional hypertensive spikes that may reach emergency levels, a normotensive state with sudden striking blood-pressure elevations that can be brief. Orthostatic hypotension is found in >50% of patients with pheochromocytoma; thus, when orthostatic hypotension presents on a background of hypertension, pheochromocytoma should be a strong diagnostic consideration.

The symptoms that accompany a pheochromocytoma-related hypertensive crisis include dizziness, flushing, visual disturbances, panic and/or anxiety, nausea, vomiting, or an epileptic aura. Although such symptoms are not completely diagnostic of pheochromocytoma, they differ sufficiently from nonendocrine hypertensive crises to merit a work-up for pheochromocytoma. Hypertensive crises are truly random in this disease. They can be set off by inadvertent manipulation of the tumor as can occur upon physical examination, exercise, postural change, micturition, and/or when eating.

An array of diseases can masquerade as a pheochromocytoma, making its diagnosis more obscure; however, about 5% of all incidentalomas are pheochromocytomas, with about 25% of all pheochromocytomas now discovered incidentally during imaging studies for unrelated disorders. Some of the more important disease imitators in this regard include menopausal syndrome, paroxysmal vasodilating headaches, postural orthostatic tachycardia syndrome, autonomic dysfunction, anxiety and/or panic disorders, acute hypoglycemia, coronary artery disease (CAD) (occult or otherwise), the use of sympathomimetic agents, ie, cocaine, and an entity termed pseudopheochromocytoma. In the case of pseudopheochromocytoma, pheochromocytoma has been ruled out and an augmented blood-pressure response to changes in the sympathoneural release of norepinephrine exists.

7. *How does CKD affect resistant hypertension?*

CKD is both a cause and a consequence of hypertension. Extracellular volume expansion is an important, if not the most important, contributing factor to the hypertension seen in CKD, and, thus, diuretic therapy plays a critical role in the treatment of CKD patients. Beyond plasma-volume expansion, CKD-related hypertension is without truly defining characteristics; consequently, the sequencing of antihypertensive medications for the CKD patient with hypertension can be arbitrary as long as diuretic therapy is begun early in the course of therapy.

In addition to its association with hypertension, CKD also affects the pharmacokinetics (and thus the duration and extent of drug response) of many of the antihypertensive medications, eg, ACE inhibitors, certain β-blockers, most diuretics. Renally cleared compounds will progressively accumulate (with repetitive dosing) at glomerular filtration rate (GFR) values <60 mL/min. Whether or not an antihypertensive compound accumulates is of some importance to the CKD patient. First, if the compound administered has a narrow therapeutic window, even moderate accumulation can move drug levels into a potentially detrimental range. For instance, accumulation of renally cleared ACE inhibitors can excessively reduce blood pressure. If the GFR were to fall with such a drop in blood pressure, ACE inhibitor clearance would drop off and blood pressure would drop even more as the drug continued to accumulate. If a compound has well-established, concentration-related side effects, they will occur more often and with possibly greater severity in the face of drug accumulation. This would be the case with renally cleared β-blockers (ie, atenolol [Tenormin®], nadolol [Corgard®]) and central nervous system (CNS) side effects. Finally, drug accumulation increases the chance of drug/drug interactions, and, in that way, creates an unnecessary therapeutic risk.

Dose adjustment of antihypertensive medications in the patient with a reduced GFR may proceed along several pathways. To maintain a therapeutic drug level for a renally cleared compound in a patient with reduced renal function, the maintenance dose may be decreased or the time interval between doses lengthened. On a practical basis, the former is more often the approach taken. Of note, in CKD drugs, ie, ACE inhibitors (primarily renally cleared compounds), are dosed to effect; thus, although prescribing information suggests that these drugs be dose adjusted in moderate-to-severe CKD, it is unusual for such changes to be applied.

Antihypertensive medications are used in the CKD patient for many reasons. First, reducing blood pressure slows the rate of progression of CKD, which seems to occur irrespective of the medication class used. Second, certain antihypertensive compounds, ie, ACE inhibitors, ARBs, have an antiproteinuric effect, which is in excess of what blood-pressure reduction alone can achieve. Third, certain antihypertensive compounds, ie, ACE inhibitors, ARBs, also provide some measure of cardiovascular protection, which is an important feature because patients with CKD maintain a high cardiovascular event-rate that spans the entire spectrum of CKD.

8. Are mood disorders associated with resistant hypertension?

A blood-pressure (and pulse-rate) measurement obtained during a panic attack will typically be elevated and often exceedingly so. Panic disorders in hypertensive patients present as sudden discrete episodes of flushing, trembling, paresthesias, sweating, and dizziness. These attacks are recurrent, may awaken the person from sleep, and are associated with anticipatory anxiety regarding a next attack. Hyperventilation is an important additional feature of panic disorder, which can separately increase blood pressure.

These patients frequently go to emergency rooms. In an unstructured environment like an emergency room, apprehension about missing a pheochromocytoma prompts what is in most instances pointless testing. In fact, studies investigating patients for pheochromocytoma have shown that as many as two thirds of these patients met criteria for either current or lifetime panic disorder. Panic disorder patients also tend to be chronically overmedicated with antihypertensive therapy, which will result in their blood-pressure levels being excessively reduced during the periods between panic attacks. While a diagnosis of panic disorder may precede one of hypertension, it is more common for panic disorder to follow the diagnosis of hypertension by virtue of a 'labeling' effect that unleashes latent tendencies to panic.

Intolerance to multiple antihypertensive drugs, particularly nondrug-specific intolerance, is commonly associated with panic disorder, anxiety, and depression. Panic disorders are thought to make hypertension more resistant to drug treatment, although this association may actually be an issue of incorrect therapies being chosen. Panic disorder/hypertension responds to selective serotonin reuptake inhibitors (SSRIs), tricyclic antidepressants (TCAs), and, for immediate symptomatic relief, alprazolam (Niravam™, Xanax®, Xanax XR®). In addition, patients should be weaned from a repetitive and impending doom pattern that arises with excessive blood-pressure monitoring at home. In many instances, abandoning home blood-pressure monitoring is an important component of treatment.

After controlling for age and gender, about 9% of adults with hypertension experienced major depression in 1999. Depression predicts a future occurrence of hypertension in normotensive subjects and increased mortality in older adults with moderate hypertension independent of other known cardiovascular risk factors. Depression can also make blood pressure resistant to therapy, if coupled with a high anxiety component, weight gain, and/or sleep disorders. Alternatively, if depression is accompanied by significant weight loss, this may decrease blood pressure and/or the need for medication. Finally, depression has been associated with medication noncompliance. In ordinary practice, newly prescribed antihypertensive medications are often quickly stopped, and adverse side effects are usually the cause. It is not uncommon in the patient with multiple nonspecific antihypertensive medication intolerances to have various psychiatric morbidities as the basis. Newer agents, ie, SSRIs, are better tolerated than older agents, ie, TCAs. However, many of the medications now commonly used in psychiatry and neurology lead to weight gain, which should be a consideration in the patient with both hypertension and depression.

9. What is the best way to determine if renal artery stenosis is the cause of resistant hypertension?

Renovascular disease clusters at the extremes of age, at least as it relates to the age of onset of hypertension. If the initial diagnosis of hypertension in an adult (particularly in a nonobese white female without a family history of hypertension) is made prior to the age 30, it is not infrequently due to fibromuscular dysplasia; whereas, new-onset hypertension in a patient >55 years should raise the possibility of atherosclerotic renal artery stenosis, particularly if the patient is a heavy smoker. Accelerated or resistant hypertension frequently is the reason for a renal artery stenosis diagnostic evaluation. 'Flash' pulmonary edema (unrelated to active ischemic heart disease) in association with sudden blood-pressure surges also can be a marker of underlying renal artery stenosis.

In general, a physical examination is of limited diagnostic help in the detection of renal artery stenosis. Evidence of multi-organ arterial disease increases the likelihood of renal artery stenosis because of the widespread nature of atheromatous changes. An epigastric-machinery-type systolic/diastolic bruit is most suggestive of renal artery stenosis. Steadily progressive azotemia (with a normal urine sediment) despite 'normal' blood-pressure readings suggests hemodynamically significant renal artery stenosis. Numerous reports also suggest that patients who develop acute renal failure while receiving diuretics and/or

ACE inhibitors have bilateral renal artery stenosis or the same in a solitary kidney. Spontaneous hypokalemia and unexplained nephrotic-range proteinuria can occasionally be seen with renal arterial disease when the RAAS is highly activated.

The ideal imaging procedure to identify renal artery stenosis should clearly show the main renal arteries and accessory or polar vessels, verify the hemodynamic significance of the lesion, locate the site of stenosis or disease, and distinguish the related pathology (ie, aneurysmal disease and/or renal masses) that may have some bearing on the treatment of this disease. In patients with indications of renovascular disease, a captopril (Capoten®)-enhanced radionuclide renal scan, duplex Doppler flow studies, and magnetic resonance angiography (MRA) provide a full complement of noninvasive and sensitive screening tests.

When an ACE inhibitor, ie, captopril (25 to 50 mg to be taken 1 hour before scanning), is combined with isotope renography, there is a noteworthy improvement in the sensitivity and specificity of radionuclide imaging, especially in the instance of unilateral renal artery stenosis (about a 30% drop in the stenotic kidney's GFR). Patients with unilateral disease and normal renal function are most suitable for a captopril renogram. The presence of either significant renal failure and/or bilateral renal artery stenosis can lessen the accuracy of captopril renography (patients with serum-creatinine values >2.5 mg/dL are often excluded). The captopril renogram was once considered the noninvasive diagnostic test of choice for patients with renal artery stenosis, but it is now consigned to a second-tier position among screening modalities because of the increased availability of duplex ultrasound and MRA.

Duplex ultrasonography combines B-mode ultrasound and Doppler examination and is a serviceable test to identify renal artery stenosis, in part, based upon cost. It provides useful information about the degree of stenosis, kidney size (and number), and other associated disease processes (eg, aneurysms, obstructions). Despite these advantages, the use of duplex Doppler ultrasonography as a screening tool is limited because of its operator dependency. MRA provides excellent imaging of the abdominal vasculature and associated anatomical structures. Contrast-enhanced MRA also provides a superior quality study when compared with noncontrast studies. Gadolinium chelate is the contrast agent of choice in patients without renal insufficiency. However, in patients with renal insufficiency, gadolinium use carries the risk of causing the damaging skin disease (called either nephrogenic systemic fibrosis or nephrogenic fibrosing dermopathy).

MRA, the 'gold' standard for arterial imaging, should be reserved for patients with an established diagnosis and indications to proceed with percutaneous transluminal angioplasty (PTA) and stenting. Renal angiography carries a small risk of radiocontrast-induced acute renal failure or atheroembolic disease particularly in patients with pre-existing renal failure and, in the case of atheroembolic disease, extensive vascular disease.

Because renal artery stenosis is commonly seen in patients with CAD, some cardiologists perform an aortogram on the 'way out' after completing a cardiac catheterization, which adds additional time and contrast to the procedure; but the quality of such images is often suboptimal. In most case, knowing the patient has renal artery stenosis adds little to the patient's overall management other than to entice the angiographer to stent the lesion in the absence of customary clinical indications.

10. What are effective drug combinations for the patient with resistant hypertension?

The effective treatment of hypertension usually requires multidrug therapy. The multidrug combinations that dominate clinical practice typically include a thiazide diuretic combined with either an ACE inhibitor, an ARB, or a β-blocker. However, there are several other medications (when added to conventional regimens) that result in an incremental reduction in blood pressure that all too often go underappreciated as to their effectiveness. Such drug combinations include a thiazide diuretic with a CCB, utilizing two CCBs from different classes, adding a peripheral β-blocker to an ACE inhibitor or a CCB, and adding an ARA or nitrates to any of several other drug classes.

Two of these drug combinations warrant particular attention. First, a pharmacokinetic interaction is an important contributing feature to the additive response of different CCB subclasses. Drugs, ie, diltiazem (Cardizem®, Cartia XT®, Diltzac®, Tiazac®), verapamil (Calan®, Covera-HS®, Isoptin® SR, Verelan®), inhibit the cytochrome P450 (CYP450) system biotransformation of a number of drugs including dihydropyridine CCBs (DCCBs), ie, amlodipine (Norvasc®), felodipine (Plendil®), isradipine (DynaCirc CR®). In principle, the interaction between verapamil or diltiazem and a DCCB can be exploited to better treat the hypertensive patient, which occurs when diltiazem or verapamil slows the metabolism of a DCCB and the resultant increase in blood levels further reduces blood pressure.

Isosorbide dinitrate (Dilatrate®-SR, Isordil®) has been shown to produce an additive anitihypertensive effect when combined with ACE inhibitors, ARBs, β-blockers, CCBs, or diuretics. For example, in a select group of patients receiving two to four conventional antihypertensive agents plus extended-release isosorbide dinitrate, the nitrate was found to further reduce blood pressure by 16 mm Hg at peak effect. If isosorbide dinitrate is chronically administered on a once-daily basis, nitrate tolerance for systolic blood-pressure reduction does not appear to occur. When sustained-release isosorbide dinitrate is considered for therapy in the patient with systolic-predominant forms of hypertension, a starting dose of 30 to 60 mg can be given once daily in the morning hours with dose titration occurring quickly thereafter.

Suggested Readings

Calhoun DA, Jones D, Textor S, et al: Resistant hypertension: diagnosis, evaluation, and treatment: a scientific statement from the American Heart Association Professional Education Committee of the Council for High Blood Pressure Research. *Circulation* 2008;117:e510-e526.

Campese VM, Mitra N, Sandee D: Hypertension in renal parenchymal disease: why is it so resistant to treatment? *Kidney Int* 2006;69:967-973.

Esler M, Schwarz R: Management of hypertension complicated by psychiatric comorbidity. *J Clin Hypertens (Greenwich)* 2007;9: 708-713.

Flack JM: Noninvasive hemodynamic measurements: an important advance in individualizing drug therapies for hypertensive patients. *Hypertension* 2006;47:646-647.

Gyamlani G, Geraci SA: Secondary hypertension due to drugs and toxins. *South Med J* 2007;100:692-699.

Hirsch S: A different approach to resistant hypertension. *Cleve Clin J Med* 2007;74:449-456.

Lenders JW, Eisenhofer G, Mannelli M, et al: Phaeochromocytoma. *Lancet* 2005;366:665-675.

Moser M, Setaro JF: Clinical practice. Resistant or difficult-to-control hypertension. *N Engl J Med* 2006;355:385-392.

Sica DA: Novel combinations in the treatment of hypertension. *Minerva Urol Nefrol* 2005;57:129-139.

Textor SC: Atherosclerotic renal artery stenosis: how big is the problem and what happens if nothing is done? *J Hypertens Suppl* 2005;23:S5-S13.

Wolk R, Shamsuzzaman AS, Somers VK: Obesity, sleep apnea, and hypertension. *Hypertension* 2003;42:1067-1074.

Appendix

Suggested Readings

Abe K, Tsuda M, Hayashi H, et al: Diagnostic usefulness of post-exercise systolic blood pressure response for detection of coronary artery disease in patients with electrocardiographic left ventricular hypertrophy. *Am J Cardiol* 1995;76:892-895.

Acanfora D, De Caprio L, Cuomo S, et al: Diagnostic value of the ratio of recovery systolic blood pressure to peak exercise systolic blood pressure for the detection of coronary artery disease. *Circulation* 1988;77:1306-1310.

Agodoa LY, Appel L, Bakris GL, et al: Effect of ramipril vs amlodipine on renal outcomes in hypertensive nephrosclerosis: a randomized controlled trial. *JAMA* 2001;285:2719-2728.

Ajisaka R, Watanabe S, Masuoka T, et al: The significance of abnormal systolic blood pressure response during supine ergometer exercise and postexercise in ischemic heart disease, studied by exercise radionuclide ventriculography. *Jpn Heart J* 1989;30:163-179.

Allison TG, Cordeiro MA, Miller TD, et al: Prognostic significance of exercise-induced systemic hypertension in healthy subjects. *Am J Cardiol* 1999;83:371-375.

Amon KW, Richards KL, Crawford MH: Usefulness of the postexercise response of systolic blood pressure in the diagnosis of coronary artery disease. *Circulation* 1984;70:951-956.

Atkins RC, Briganti EM, Lewis JB, et al: Proteinuria reduction and progression to renal failure in patients with type 2 diabetes mellitus and overt nephropathy. *Am J Kidney Dis* 2005;45:281-287.

Azor receives FDA approval for treatment of high blood pressure. *FDA Drug Approvals*. Available at: http://www.drugs.com/newdrugs/azor-receives-fda-approval-blood-pressure-655.html. Accessed September 11, 2008.

Bakris GL, Weir MR: Angiotensin-converting enzyme inhibitor-associated elevations in serum creatinine: is this a cause for concern? *Arch Intern Med* 2000;160:685-693.

Bakris GL, Weir MR, Secic M, et al: Differential effects of calcium antagonist subclasses on markers of nephropathy progression. *Kidney Int* 2004;65:1991-2002.

Bakris GL, Williams M, Dworkin L, et al: Preserving renal function in adults with hypertension and diabetes: a consensus approach. National Kidney Foundation Hypertension and Diabetes Executive Committees Working Group. *Am J Kidney Dis* 2000;36:646-661.

Bangalore S, Kamalakkannan G, Parkar S, et al: Fixed-dose combinations improve medication compliance: a meta-analysis. *Am J Med* 2007;120:713-719.

Bangalore S, Messerli FH, Kostis JB, et al: Cardiovascular protection using beta-blockers: a critical review of the evidence. *J Am Coll Cardiol* 2007;50:563-572.

Barnett AH, Bain SC, Bouter P, et al: Angiotensin-receptor blockade versus converting-enzyme inhibition in type 2 diabetes and nephropathy. *N Engl J Med* 2004;351:1952-1961.

Beckett NS, Peters R, Fletcher AE, et al, and the HYVET Study Group: Treatment of hypertension in patients 80 years of age or older. *N Engl J Med* 2008;358:1887-1898.

Bradley HA, Wiysonge CS, Volmink JA, et al: How strong is the evidence for use of beta-blockers as first-line therapy for hypertension? Systematic review and meta-analysis. *J Hypertens* 2006;24:2131-2141.

Brenner BM, Cooper ME, de Zeeuw D, et al: Effects of losartan on renal and cardiovascular outcomes in patients with type 2 diabetes and nephropathy. *N Engl J Med* 2001;345:861-869.

Brewster LM, van Montfrans GA, Kleijnen J: Systematic review: antihypertensive drug therapy in black patients. *Ann Intern Med* 2004;141:614-627.

Brodde OE, Kroemer HK: Drug-drug interactions of beta-adrenoceptor blockers. *Arzneimittelforschung* 2003;53:814-822.

Brown MJ: Aliskiren. *Circulation* 2008;118:773-784.

Bucca CB, Brussino L, Battisti A, et al: Diuretics in obstructive sleep apnea with diastolic heart failure. *Chest* 2007;132:440-446.

Calhoun DA, Jones D, Textor S, et al: Resistant hypertension: diagnosis, evaluation, and treatment: a scientific statement from the American Heart Association Professional Education Committee of the Council for High Blood Pressure Research. *Circulation* 2008;117:e510-e526.

Calhoun DA: Low-dose aldosterone blockade as a new treatment paradigm for controlling resistant hypertension. *J Clin Hypertens (Greenwich)* 2007;9(1 suppl 1):19-24.

Campese VM, Mitra N, Sandee D: Hypertension in renal parenchymal disease: why is it so resistant to treatment? *Kidney Int* 2006;69:967-973.

Carter BL, Sica DA: Strategies to improve the cardiovascular risk profile of thiazide-type diuretics as used in the management of hypertension. *Expert Opin Drug Saf* 2007;6:583-594.

Casas JP, Chua W, Loukogeorgakis S, et al: Effect of inhibitors of the renin-angiotensin system and other antihypertensive drugs on renal outcomes: systematic review and meta-analysis. *Lancet* 2005;366:2026-2033.

Chrostowska M, Szczech R, Narkiewicz K: Antihypertensive therapy in the obese hypertensive patient. *Curr Opin Nephrol Hypertens* 2006;15:487-492.

Cicolin A, Mangiardi L, Mutani R, et al: Angiotensin-converting enzyme inhibitors and obstructive sleep apnea. *Mayo Clin Proc* 2006;81:53-55.

Cutler JA, Davis BR: Thiazide-type diuretics and beta-adrenergic blockers as first-line drug treatments for hypertension. *Circulation* 2008;117:2691-2704.

de Zeeuw D, Remuzzi G, Parving HH, et al: Proteinuria, a target for renoprotection in patients with type 2 diabetic nephropathy: lessons from RENAAL. *Kidney Int* 2004;65:2309-2320.

de Zeeuw D, Remuzzi G, Parving HH, et al: Albuminuria, a therapeutic target for cardiovascular protection in type 2 diabetic patients with nephropathy. *Circulation* 2004;110:921-927.

Drukteinis JS, Roman MJ, Fabsitz RR, et al: Cardiac and systemic hemodynamic characteristics of hypertension and prehypertension in adolescents and young adults: the Strong Heart Study. *Circulation* 2007;115:221-227.

Dzau VJ, Bernstein K, Celermajer D, et al: The relevance of tissue angiotensin-converting enzyme: manifestations in mechanistic and endpoint data. *Am J Cardiol* 2001;88:1L-20L.

Effects of calcium antagonists on the risks of coronary heart disease, cancer and bleeding. Ad Hoc Subcommittee of the Liaison Committee of the World Health Organisation and the International Society of Hypertension. *J Hum Hypertens* 1997;11:331-342.

Eijkelkamp WB, Zhang Z, Remuzzi G, et al: Albuminuria is a target for renoprotective therapy independent from blood pressure in patients with type 2 diabetic nephropathy: post hoc analysis from the Reduction of Endpoints in NIDDM with the Angiotensin II Antagonist Losartan (RENAAL) trial. *J Am Soc Nephrol* 2007;18:1540-1546.

Ernst ME, Carter BL, Goerdt CJ, et al: Comparative antihypertensive effects of hydrochlorothiazide and chlorthalidone on ambulatory and office blood pressure. *Hypertension* 2006;47:352-358.

Ersoy A, Kahvecioglu S, Ersoy C, et al: Anemia due to losartan in hypertensive renal transplant recipients without posttransplant erythrocytosis. *Transplant Proc* 2005;37:2148-2150.

Esler M, Schwarz R: Management of hypertension complicated by psychiatric comorbidity. *J Clin Hypertens (Greenwich)* 2007;9:708-713.

Exforge receives final US approval as new and powerful treatment option for patients with high blood pressure. *FDA Drug Approvals.* Available at: http://www.drugs.com/newdrugs/exforge-receives-final-us-approval-new-powerful-option-patients-blood-pressure-535.html. Accessed September 11, 2008.

Ferdinand KC: Hypertension in minority populations. *J Clin Hypertens (Greenwich)* 2006;8:365-368.

Flack JM: Noninvasive hemodynamic measurements: an important advance in individualizing drug therapies for hypertensive patients. *Hypertension* 2006;47:646-647.

Fleisher LA, Beckman JA, Brown KA, et al: ACC/AHA 2006 guideline update on perioperative cardiovascular evaluation for noncardiac surgery: focused update on perioperative beta-blocker therapy: a report of the American College of Cardiology/American Heart Association Task Force on Practice Guidelines (Writing Committee to Update the 2002 Guidelines on Perioperative Cardiovascular Evaluation for Noncardiac Surgery): developed in collaboration with the American Society of Echocardiography, American Society of Nuclear Cardiology, Heart Rhythm Society, Society of Cardiovascular Anesthesiologists, Society for Cardiovascular Angiography and Interventions, and Society for Vascular Medicine and Biology. *Circulation* 2006;113:2662-2674.

Fletcher GF, Balady GJ, Amsterdam EA, et al: Exercise standards for testing and training: a statement for healthcare professionals from the American Heart Association. *Circulation* 2001;104:1694-1740.

Fogari R, Zoppi A: Effects of antihypertensive therapy on sexual activity in hypertensive men. *Curr Hypertens Rep* 2002;4:202-210.

Frishman WH, Alwarshetty M: Beta-adrenergic blockers in systemic hypertension: pharmacokinetic considerations related to the current guidelines. *Clin Pharmacokinet* 2002;41:505-516.

Frishman WH, Bryzinski BS, Coulson LR, et al: A multifactorial trial design to assess combination therapy in hypertension. Treatment with bisoprolol and hydrochlorothiazide. *Arch Intern Med* 1994; 154:1461-1468.

Garg R, Yusuf S: Overview of randomized trials of angiotensin-converting enzyme inhibitors on mortality and morbidity in patients with heart failure. Collaborative Group on ACE Inhibitor Trials. *JAMA* 1995;273:1450-1456.

Garthwaite SM, McMahon EG: The evolution of aldosterone antagonists. *Mol Cell Endocrinol* 2004;217:27-31.

Giles T, Aranda JM Jr, Suh DC, et al: Ethnic/racial variations in blood pressure awareness, treatment, and control. *J Clin Hypertens (Greenwich)* 2007;9:345-354.

Goel R, Majeed F, Vogel R, et al: Exercise-induced hypertension, endothelial dysfunction, and coronary artery disease in a marathon runner. *Am J Cardiol* 2007;99:743-744.

Goncalves SC, Martinez D, Gus M, et al: Obstructive sleep apnea and resistant hypertension: a case-control study. *Chest* 2007;132: 1858-1862.

Gradman AH, Kad R: Renin inhibition in hypertension. *J Am Coll Cardiol* 2008;51:519-528.

Gyamlani G, Geraci SA: Secondary hypertension due to drugs and toxins. *South Med J* 2007;100:692-699.

Haentjens P, Van Meerhaeghe A, Moscariello A, et al: The impact of continuous positive airway pressure on blood pressure in patients with obstructive sleep apnea syndrome: evidence from a meta-analysis of placebo-controlled randomized trials. *Arch Intern Med* 2007;167:757-764.

Hart PD, Bakris GL: Should beta-blockers be used to control hypertension in people with chronic kidney disease? *Semin Nephrol* 2007;27:555-564.

Hirsch S: A different approach to resistant hypertension. *Cleve Clin J Med* 2007;74:449-456.

Jamerson K, DeQuattro V: The impact of ethnicity on response to antihypertensive therapy. *Am J Med* 1996;101:22S-32S.

Jamerson KA, Bakris GL, Wun CC, et al: Rationale and design of the avoiding cardiovascular events through combination therapy in patients living with systolic hypertension (ACCOMPLISH) trial: the first randomized controlled trial to compare the clinical outcome effects of first-line combination therapies in hypertension. *Am J Hypertens* 2004;17:793-801.

Johnson BF, Saunders R, Hickler R, et al: The effects of thiazide diuretics upon plasma lipoproteins. *J Hypertens* 1986;4:235-239.

Jurva JW, Phillips SA, Syed AQ, et al: The effect of exertional hypertension evoked by weight lifting on vascular endothelial function. *J Am Coll Cardiol* 2006;48:588-589.

Kuniyoshi FH, Somers VK: Sleep apnea in hypertension: when, how, and why should we treat? *Hypertension* 2006;47:818-819.

Law MR, Wald NJ, Morris JK, et al: Value of low dose combination treatment with blood pressure lowering drugs: analysis of 354 randomised trials. *BMJ* 2003;326:1427.

Lenders JW, Eisenhofer G, Mannelli M, et al: Phaeochromocytoma. *Lancet* 2005;366:665-675.

Leslie WS, Hankey CR, Lean ME: Weight gain as an adverse effect of some commonly prescribed drugs: a systematic review. *QJM* 2007;100:395-404.

Lewis EJ, Hunsicker LG, Clarke WR, et al, and Collaborative Study Group: Renoprotective effect of the angiotensin-receptor antagonist irbesartan in patients with nephropathy due to type 2 diabetes. *N Engl J Med* 2001;345:851-860.

Liew D, Krum H: Aldosterone receptor antagonists for hypertension: what do they offer? *Drugs* 2003;63:1963-1972.

Mancia G, Grassi G, Zanchetti A: New-onset diabetes and antihypertensive drugs. *J Hypertens* 2006;24:3-10.

Margolis KL, Piller LB, Ford CE, et al: Blood pressure control in Hispanics in the antihypertensive and lipid-lowering treatment to prevent heart attack trial. *Hypertension* 2007;50:854-861.

Materson BJ, Reda DJ, Cushman WC, et al: Single-drug therapy for hypertension in men. A comparison of six antihypertensive agents with placebo. The Department of Veterans Affairs Cooperative Study Group on Antihypertensive Agents. *N Engl J Med* 1993;328: 914-921.

McMurray J, Pitt B, Latini R, et al: Effects of the oral direct renin inhibitor aliskiren in patients with symptomatic heart failure. *Circulation: Heart Failure* 2008;1:17-24.

Messerli FH, Bangalore S, Julius S: Risk/benefit assessment of beta-blockers and diuretics precludes their use for first-line therapy in hypertension. *Circulation* 2008;117:2706-2715.

Mokhlesi B, Tulaimat A: Recent advances in obesity hypoventilation syndrome. *Chest* 2007;132:1322-1336.

Moser M, Setaro JF: Clinical practice. Resistant or difficult-to-control hypertension. *N Engl J Med* 2006;355:385-392.

Narva AS: The spectrum of kidney disease in American Indians. *Kidney Int Suppl* 2003;83:S3-S7.

Neutel JM, Black HR, Weber MA: Combination therapy with diuretics: an evolution of understanding. *Am J Med* 1996;101(3A):61S-70S.

Nishizaka MK, Zaman MA, Calhoun DA: Efficacy of low-dose spironolactone in subjects with resistant hypertension. *Am J Hypertens* 2003;16(11 pt 1):925-930.

ONTARGET Investigators and Yusuf S, Teo KK, Pogue J, et al: Telmisartan, ramipril, or both in patients at high risk for vascular events. *N Engl J Med* 2008;358:1547-1559.

Palatini P, Benetos A, Julius S: Impact of increased heart rate on clinical outcomes in hypertension: implications for antihypertensive drug therapy. *Drugs* 2006;66:133-144.

Park IU, Taylor AL: Race and ethnicity in trials of antihypertensive therapy to prevent cardiovascular outcomes: a systematic review. *Ann Fam Med* 2007;5:444-452.

Parving HH, Lehnert H, Brochner-Mortensen J, et al: The effect of irbesartan on the development of diabetic nephropathy in patients with type 2 diabetes. *N Engl J Med* 2001;345:870-878.

Parving HH, Persson F, Lewis JB, et al, and AVOID Study Investigators: Aliskiren combined with losartan in type 2 diabetes and nephropathy. *N Engl J Med* 2008;358:2433-2446.

Pedersen ME, Cockcroft JR: The vasodilatory beta-blockers. *Curr Hypertens Rep* 2007;9:269-277.

Pickering TG, Miller NH, Ogedegbe G, et al: Call to action on use and reimbursement for home blood pressure monitoring: executive summary: a joint scientific statement from the American Heart Association, American Society Of Hypertension, and Preventive Cardiovascular Nurses Association. *Hypertension* 2008;52:1-9.

Piepho RW, Culbertson VL, Rhodes RS: Drug interactions with the calcium-entry blockers. *Circulation* 1987;75(6 pt 2):V181-V194.

Pohl MA, Blumenthal S, Cordonnier DJ, et al: Independent and additive impact of blood pressure control and angiotensin II receptor blockade on renal outcomes in the irbesartan diabetic nephropathy trial: clinical implications and limitations. *J Am Soc Nephrol* 2005;16:3027-3037.

Pratt-Ubunama MN, Nishizaka MK, Boedefeld RL, et al: Plasma aldosterone is related to severity of obstructive sleep apnea in subjects with resistant hypertension. *Chest* 2007;131:453-459.

Prisant LM, Dillard TA, Blanchard AR: Obstructive sleep apnea syndrome. *J Clin Hypertens (Greenwich)* 2006;8:746-750.

Psaty B, Smith N, Siscovick D, et al: Health outcomes associated with antihypertensive therapies used as first-line agents: A systematic review and meta-analysis. *JAMA* 1997;277:739-745.

Rahmouni K, Correia ML, Haynes WG, et al: Obesity-associated hypertension: new insights into mechanisms. *Hypertension* 2005;45:9-14.

Reyes AJ: Cardiovascular drugs and serum uric acid. *Cardiovasc Drugs Ther* 2003;17:397-414.

Rose LI, Underwood RH, Newmark SR, et al: Pathophysiology of spironolactone-induced gynecomastia. *Ann Int Med* 1977;87: 398-403.

Santos J, Planas R, Pardo A, et al: Spironolactone alone or in combination with furosemide in the treatment of moderate ascites in nonazotemic cirrhosis. A randomized comparative study of efficacy and safety. *J Hepatol* 2003;39:187-192.

Saunders E, Weir MR, Kong BW, et al: A comparison of the efficacy and safety of a beta-blocker, a calcium channel blocker, and a converting enzyme inhibitor in hypertensive blacks. *Arch Intern Med* 1990;150:1707-1713.

Schjoedt KJ, Rossing K, Juhl TR, et al: Beneficial impact of spironolactone in diabetic nephropathy. *Kidney Int* 2005;68:2829-2836.

Schmieder RE, Hilgers KF, Schlaich MP, et al: Renin-angiotensin system and cardiovascular risk. *Lancet* 2007;369:1208-1219.

Schoolwerth AC, Sica DA, Ballermann BJ, et al: Renal considerations in angiotensin converting enzyme inhibitor therapy: a statement for healthcare professionals from the Council on the Kidney in Cardiovascular Disease and the Council for High Blood Pressure Research of the American Heart Association. *Circulation* 2001;104:1985-1991.

Schrier RW, Estacio RO, Esler A, et al: Effects of aggressive blood pressure control in normotensive type 2 diabetic patients on albuminuria, retinopathy and strokes. *Kidney Int* 2002;61:1086-1097.

Sever P: The heterogeneity of hypertension: why doesn't every patient respond to every antihypertensive drug? *J Hum Hypertens* 1995;9(suppl 2):S33-S36.

Sica DA: Novel combinations in the treatment of hypertension. *Minerva Urol Nefrol* 2005;57:129-139.

Sica DA: Pharmacokinetics and pharmacodynamics of mineralocorticoid blocking agents and their effects on potassium homeostasis. *Heart Fail Rev* 2005;10:23-29.

Sica DA: Diuretic-related side effects: development and treatment. *J Clin Hypertens (Greenwich)* 2004;6:532-540.

Sica DA: Angiotensin-converting enzyme inhibitors side effects—physiologic and non-physiologic considerations. *J Clin Hypertens (Greenwich)* 2004;6:410-416.

Sica DA: Rationale for fixed-dose combinations in the treatment of hypertension: the cycle repeats. *Drugs* 2002;62:443-462.

Sica DA: Current concepts of pharmacotherapy in hypertension—ophthalmically administered beta blockers and their cardiopulmonary effects. *J Clin Hypertens (Greenwich)* 2001;3:175-178.

Sica DA, Black HR: Current concepts of pharmacotherapy in hypertension: ACE inhibitor-related angioedema: can angiotensin-receptor blockers be safely used? *J Clin Hypertens (Greenwich)* 2002;4:375-380.

Sica DA, Hess M: Pharmacotherapy in congestive heart failure: aldosterone receptor antagonism: interface with hyperkalemia in heart failure. *Congest Heart Fail* 2004;10:259-264.

Sim JJ, Rasgon SA, Derose SF: Sleep apnea and hypertension: prevalence in chronic kidney disease. *J Clin Hypertens (Greenwich)* 2007;9:837-841.

Srinath Reddy K, Shah B, Varghese C, et al: Responding to the threat of chronic diseases in India. *Lancet* 2005;366:1744-1749.

Stewart KJ, Ouyang P, Bacher AC, et al: Exercise effects on cardiac size and left ventricular diastolic function: relationships to changes in fitness, fatness, blood pressure and insulin resistance. *Heart* 2006;92:893-898.

Strom BL, Schinnar R, Apter AJ, et al: Absence of cross-reactivity between sulfonamide antibiotics and sulfonamide nonantibiotics. *N Engl J Med* 2003;349:1628-1635.

Syme AN, Blanchard BE, Guidry MA, et al: Peak systolic blood pressure on a graded maximal exercise test and the blood pressure response to an acute bout of submaximal exercise. *Am J Cardiol* 2006;98:938-943.

Taylor AJ, Beller GA: Postexercise systolic blood pressure response: association with the presence and extent of perfusion abnormalities on thallium-201 scintigraphy. *Am Heart J* 1995;129:227-234.

The Telmisartan Randomised AssessmeNt Study in ACE iNtolerant subjects with cardiovascular Disease (TRANSCEND) Investigators: Effects of the angiotensin-receptor blocker telmisartan on cardiovascular events in high-risk patients intolerant to angiotensin-converting enzyme inhibitors: a randomised controlled trial. *Lancet* 2008 Aug 29;Epub ahead of publication.

Textor SC: Atherosclerotic renal artery stenosis: how big is the problem and what happens if nothing is done? *J Hypertens Suppl* 2005;23:S5-S13.

Tsuda M, Hatano K, Hayashi H, et al: Diagnostic value of postexercise systolic blood pressure response for detecting coronary artery disease in patients with or without hypertension. *Am Heart J* 1993;125:718-725.

Waeber B: Very-low-dose combination: a first-line choice for the treatment of hypertension? *J Hypertens Suppl* 2003;21:S3-S10.

Weber MA, Ruilope L, Giles TD, et al: First-step use of fixed-dose combination treatment in stage 2 hypertensive patients: has the time come? *J Clin Hypertens (Greenwich)* 2007;9:276-284.

Weinberger MH, White WB, Ruilope LM, et al: Effects of eplerenone versus losartan in patients with low-renin hypertension. *Am Heart J* 2005;150:426-433.

Weir MR: The rationale for combination versus single-entity therapy in hypertension. *Am J Hypertens* 1998;11:163S-169S.

Wolk R, Shamsuzzaman AS, Somers VK: Obesity, sleep apnea, and hypertension. *Hypertension* 2003;42:1067-1074.

Yeates K, Tonelli M: Indigenous health: update on the impact of diabetes and chronic kidney disease. *Curr Opin Nephrol Hypertens* 2006;15:588-592.

Yusuf S, Sleight P, Pogue J, et al: Effects of an angiotensin-converting enzyme inhibitor, ramipril, on cardiovascular events in high-risk patients. The Heart Outcomes Prevention Evaluation Study Investigators. *N Engl J Med* 2000;342:145-153.

Zillich AJ, Garg J, Basu S, et al: Thiazide diuretics, potassium, and the development of diabetes: a quantitative review. *Hypertension* 2006;48:219-224.

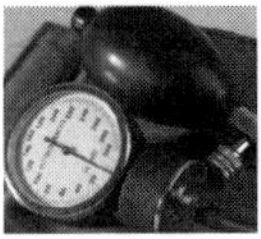

Index

A

D

E

F

G

H

I

J

K

L

M

N

O

P

Q

R

S

T

U

V

W

X

Z